Oops!

Published by

Adams Media, a division of F+W Media, Inc.

57 Littlefield Street, Avon, MA 02322. U.S.A.

www.adamsmedia.com

ISBN 10: 1-4405-6206-7

ISBN 13: 978-1-4405-6206-8

eISBN 10: 1-4405-6207-5

eISBN 13: 978-1-4405-6207-5

Printed in the United States of America.

10 9 8 7 6 5 4 3 2 1

This book is intended as general information only, and should not be used to diagnose or treat any health condition. In light of the complex, individual, and specific nature of health problems, this book is not intended to replace professional medical advice. The ideas, procedures, and suggestions in this book are intended to supplement, not replace, the advice of a trained medical professional. Consult your physician before adopting any of the suggestions in this book, as well as about any condition that may require diagnosis or medical attention. The author and publisher disclaim any liability arising directly or indirectly from the use of this book.

Many of the designations used by manufacturers and sellers to distinguish their product are claimed as trademarks. Where those designations appear in this book and F+W Media was aware of a trademark claim, the designations have been printed with initial capital letters.

Cover image © 123rf.com.

This book is available at quantity discounts for bulk purchases.
For information, please call 1-800-289-0963.

A **Positive** Guide to Your Unexpected Pregnancy

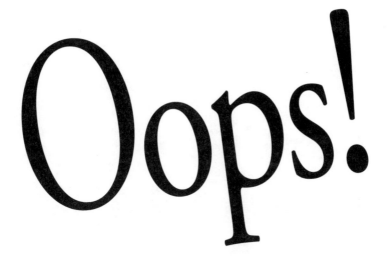

Oops!

HOW TO ROCK
THE MOTHER
OF ALL SURPRISES

TRACY MOORE
Contributor to Jezebel.com

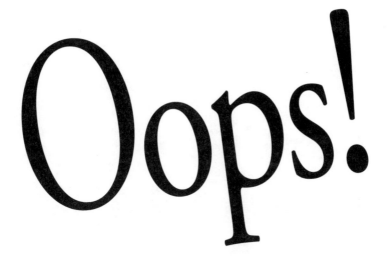
Aadamsmedia
Avon, Massachusetts

CONTENTS

Introduction ... **11**

STAGE **1:** **SHOCK . . .**
HOLY SHIT, YOU'RE PREGNANT ... 17

1. You're So Not Alone (Because There's a Baby Inside You) ... **19**

2. Did I Screw Up My Chances for a Healthy Baby? ... **25**

3. Are There Any Disadvantages to an Unplanned Pregnancy? ... **33**

4. Ten Advantages to an Unplanned Pregnancy ... **35**

5. Will My Life Be Over? ... **41**

6. But I'm Not Even a Baby Person! ... **47**

STAGE **2:** **HELP! . . .**
HOW TO DEAL WITH PREGNANCY OBSTACLES ... 51

7. What Will People Say about Me? (Because I Know They Will Say Things) ... **53**

8. If Your Friends and Family Start Acting Like Dramatic Weirdos ... **59**

9. How the Hell Do I Get Ready for an Actual Baby? ... **65**

10. How to Eat All the Stuff You Aren't Supposed To ... **75**

11. Everything Is Beautiful (in Its Own Disgusting Way): A Public Service Rant ... **81**

12. What Not to Wear, Unplanned Pregnancy Edition ... **89**

13. Your New Boyfriend: Food ... **95**

14. How to Deal with Emotional Upheaval ... **101**

STAGE 3: LOGISTICS . . . REAL-LIFE STUFF TO FIGURE OUT ... 109

15. What Will an Unplanned Baby Do to My Relationship? ... **111**

16. Working Whilst Pregnant ... **119**

17. Figuring Out Your Maternity Leave ... **127**

18. Finding Good Child Care ... **131**

19. You Are about to Lose One Precious Commodity Forever: Free Time ... **139**

20. If You're Adding to Your Brood ... **147**

21. What You Should Really Take Away from Birthing Class ... **153**

STAGE 4: EXCITEMENT . . . THE ACTUAL BABY ARRIVES! ... 161

22. The Baby Is Coming: A Few Thoughts on Labor ... **163**

23. Holy Shit, You're IN LABOR ... **171**

24. Welcome to Your New, Cliché-Ridden Life ... **177**

25. Get Used to Feeling Like Shit for a While ... **187**

26. Managing Visitors the First Few Weeks Home ... **193**

27. What to Wear Postpartum ... **199**

28. Breastfeeding: Kind of a Bitch ... **205**

STAGE 5: **ROCKING IT . . . YOUR LIFE WITH BABY ... 211**

29. The Great Baby Excuse ... **213**

30. Four Types of Women When It Comes to Post-Birth Sex ... **217**

31. How to Be Cool with a Baby ... **221**

32. Being a Mom Isn't Easy—You'll Need a Little Help from Your "Friends" ... **229**

33. All Babies Are Sweet, Precious Bundles of Joy, and Other Baby Myths ... **237**

34. Reflections ... **243**

APPENDIX: Resources ... 249

Index ... 253

For Lance and Edie

"Nearly all the best things that came to me in life have been unexpected, unplanned by me."

—Carl Sandburg

INTRODUCTION

When I found myself suddenly knocked up in the summer of 2009, my carefree life skidded to a halt. I went from being an immature, thirty-three-year-old boozehound working at an alt-weekly, hitting the bars four nights a week, to a gobsmacked puddle of Jell-O facing down the firmest adult-like deadline of my life. I may have been a grown woman with a job, a 401(k), and even a husband who was happy about being blindsided, but I felt about as emotionally qualified to have a baby as any cast member of *16 and Pregnant*.

This was, in large part, because I was one of those people who are pretty sure they aren't going to have any kids. As a result, I lived my life like someone who doesn't need to ever grow up enough to take care of a baby. I avoided pregnancy talk and babies and general nurturing so successfully that I realized I had almost no common knowledge about what pregnancy even entailed, much less how to hold, talk to, or feed an infant, or explain to one what a good rock band was. Now here I was, pregnant.

Let me say this first: Though this news was *unexpected*, it was not *unwelcome*. Yes, it would change everything. But what it did *not* change was the fact that I had no idea what the hell I was doing.

It sounds cliché (get used to that), but some of the best things in life are, indeed, random. They are the unexpected turns that yield previously unimagined fruit—the accidental meeting, the oddly timed good idea that lands just right, the decision to stick with *New Girl* after

11

its first few episodes. In fact, almost all my best memories come from events where I had no idea what would happen next—and not just because I was doing shots.

So it was with pregnancy. I could not envision the turns it would take, emotionally, physically, or emotionally. Did I mention emotionally? Not having planned this thing, I had never bothered to imagine its multitextured possibilities, much less take folic acid. But I was curious about this unknown, wildly divergent path that had sprung up before me, and a funny thing happened: In spite of intellectually not wanting to be pregnant, once I was . . . there was, for me, no going back. I was invested, and I was curious. And I was really happy (and reassured) to discover that those hardscrabble qualities will often take you farther than the best-laid plans.

"Being slightly paranoid is like being slightly pregnant—it tends to get worse."

—Molly Ivins

So I rolled with it. But that is not at all the same thing as being ready for the road ahead. And that I was not. I was amazed, though, to find a glut of information available about the physical and medical aspects of pregnancy. Seemingly endless books, websites, and forums—all in reassuringly tedious detail—covered nearly every question I could imagine about the basics of gestating, from heartburn to hemorrhoids.

What I couldn't find was anything much about the emotional chaos and confusion of an unplanned pregnancy from the perspective of an alleged adult who had zero intention of ever having a baby, especially if it meant there would be this much farting. Plus, I needed logistical guidance, stat: My husband and I didn't have the dough, the gear, or the lifestyle to bring a baby into the world. And scarier, we didn't even know what we didn't know.

What's more, what was out there about "unplanned pregnancies" seemed so academic, so antiseptic, so religious—none of it was able to help me figure out why I was suddenly reliving my shitty childhood, why the show *My Wife and Kids* was now funny to me, or how to remove five years of cat hair and cigarette funk from a sofa before a baby comes.

There was also nothing to help me quit smoking cold turkey but also not consume everything in sight like some kind of pregnant human garbage disposal. Nothing about how to keep hanging out with your friends while you're sober, especially now that they are suddenly the most annoying people in the world.

There was no warning that I might regress to the emotional state of my teenage self, but sure enough, there I was, fighting with my baby daddy, hating my mom again, and missing the best parties.

I wrote this book because it's the book I longed for when I was pregnant. Something that would take me through the logistics of how to prep for a surprise pregnancy with a limited amount of time to stockpile money and desmokify a house. A place to vent about what a pain in the ass it is to suddenly deal with a once-autonomous body that feels hijacked and smells, bewilderingly, like soup. A place to laugh about the clichéd discomforts of pregnancy from the perspective of someone who found herself there by accident.

A place that celebrates the what-the-fuckness of breeding, on purpose or not. And ultimately, a place that understands that you can loathe everything about pregnancy, from ugly maternity tops to morning sickness to swollen ankles, and yet still love the child you are growing without question, not in spite of it but because of it. Especially when the growing of that child causes you to get the weirdest, grossest ear zits imaginable.

If I have done anything correctly, I have created that space for you and every other adult woman who finds herself inexplicably knocked up and scared shitless, ready to do this thing right but kind of wishing there was a TV show called *33 and Pregnant* to take you through it.

The biggest gamble in the universe, hands down, has got to be the making of a life. But if I am proof of anything, it's that it can be done, even well. In fact, it's very similar to that E.L. Doctorow quote about writing: "It's like driving at night in the fog. You can only see as far as your headlights, but you can make the whole trip that way."

"Babies are always more trouble than you thought and more wonderful than you ever dreamed."

—Charles Osgood

So to face this thing, I suggest taking off the mask of knowing and diving to the bottom of not knowing. It's terrifying, but it might just be a once-in-a-lifetime thrill. And this is coming from a person who has sat in the backseat of a 1976 Chevelle, driving around farmland, ramming into hay bales. At night. With no headlights. For kicks. You think I don't know thrills?

Maybe you never wanted kids. Maybe you weren't sure if you wanted kids. Maybe you wanted kids but just not now, for the love of all that's holy—just *not now*. Maybe you have kids already and you thought you were "done."

But now here you are, with a bun in the oven, a bean on the sprout, an egg in the skillet. And whether you are calling it your "Oops Baby," a "Little Surprise," or your "Bonus Round," you are keeping this kid. Still, your emotions will need time to catch up. You'll realize this when your first instinct after happily announcing the news is to download a sad trombone MP3 and walk moodily around, pressing Play at random intervals.

To aid in your epic journey, I've organized this book into the five stages—Shock, Help!, Logistics, Excitement, and Rocking It—that you're likely to experience. I'll walk you through the basics: the logistics, and emotional boot camp of making your life baby-ready. Though nothing can predict exactly how or in what ways you might feel blindsided, uplifted, shocked, or awed (or all of the above, simultaneously) by this decision to breed on the fly, that moment will come, and you will wonder: What the hell have I gotten myself into?

But think of it this way. When you do not know what is coming, you cannot convincingly talk yourself out of the ride. You have to eventually just let go of the bracing fear of it all and accept the unwieldy twists and turns. So if you too have found yourself knocked up without a road map, just keep driving. Dodge the hay bales, though. And do everyone a favor—keep the lights on.

STAGE 1:

SHOCK . . . HOLY SHIT, YOU'RE PREGNANT

1.

YOU'RE SO NOT ALONE
(Because There's a Baby Inside You)

So, you're accidentally knocked up.

Surprise!

Congrats? Congrats!

You, or the judgy people around you, are probably thinking, birth control much? Pulling out? Abstinence? Anybody? Ain't no grown-ass woman got to be pregnant if she don't want, amirite?

Well . . . yes and no. And yet, according to the U.S. Centers for Disease Control and Prevention, 49 percent of pregnancies in 2011 were "mistimed, unplanned, or unwanted." Yes, really. So look around at all the children you see and know that one out of every two of those darlings is an oops, a shrug, an okay-I-guess-let's-do-this.

In other words, you're not alone. Even though you might be feeling that way and thus are considering a Thelma and Louise– or Wile E. Coyote–style move that reflects the very oh-shit feelings of this endeavor.

First, DO NOT DRIVE OFF A CLIFF. There are no jalapeño nachos down there, trust me. And unless you actually starred in *Thelma and Louise,* you didn't even just pretend-sleep with young Brad Pitt, so obviously you still have some living to do.

Second, allow me to restate the facts, or at least the only fact that matters to us: 49 percent of pregnancies are unplanned. Your situation is, in fact, totally normal. Mundane, even. It may not be anyone's ideal, but it's actually how the whole thing works about half of the freaking time. This information should be posted in bold, flashy fonts at every major intersection in the universe, such a significant fact it is. It's also kind of awesome if you think about it. Life is unpredictable. The rules are always changing. Dice! Rollin'!

Also, if you think about it, aspects of all pregnancies are unknown. Even if you always wanted kids, you still can't have much of an idea what it would really be like to have a baby, because there is no way to know what it is really like to have a baby without doing it. Even if you wanted to get pregnant, you couldn't have known exactly how your body would react to the experience. And even if you already had twelve babies, you still could not have predicted what it would be like to have this particular baby, because all babies are different.

"The condom broke. I know how stupid that sounds. It's the reproductive version of the dog ate my homework."

—Jennifer Weiner, *Little Earthquakes*

The point is, a big part of pregnancy and parenting is out of your hands, and that's not always bad. That's part of the fun, as terrifying as this may sound to you now. And try as we might to control our fates, life creeps in sometimes. Did you hear me? Life creeps in.

How would I know? Because sometimes it creeps into the middle of nowhere in rural Tennessee at the music festival Bonnaroo. Okay, so it wasn't the *middle* of nowhere, more like the middle of a somewhat concealed spot near a bunch of campers in the mud. With my husband. Who had been told by actual doctors that he was infertile.

Record scratch.

When I got pregnant in that field, my favorite pastimes included doing nothing and not having to do anything—usually while drinking and smoking, and almost always with a very bad attitude. So you can see that I was not the greatest candidate for doing a lot of stuff all at once, such as paying attention, feeding something often, and caring a lot, as one does with a baby. And at such early hours.

Moreover, when I found out I was pregnant, I had spent the weekend literally bouncing up and down on a jet ski at my friend's parents' lake house in Alabama, where we had used the majority of our time getting wasted off Miller Lite. In a can. Messing around with fireworks. Cut to next scene: I was smoking a cigarette and drinking a beer while sitting on the toilet hunched over an e.p.t. stick. Don't ask why I was doing all those things together—at the time it seemed really appropriate.

My husband and I had $90 between us. No health insurance. Two months of marriage under his honest-to-god ammo belt. (That's a belt made entirely of empty bullet cartridges that he wore onstage in his fifteen-person rock band with face paint and robots. The one that paid him in burritos.)

Did I mention we were not in our early twenties but in our late twenties? And by late twenties I mean I was actually thirty-three? Did I mentioned we owned two gray cats that shed a lot of long, fine, gray hair onto everything, and if you ran around too fast in any room it might be like a snowglobe of long, fine, gray cat hair? And that they couldn't really get all their crap into the litter box so it was on the floor *around* the litter box frequently, too? And that my diet consisted of Parliament Lights and a sack full of Krystals?

Suffice it to say I did not want a baby. Or, rather, I didn't think, for a long list of reasons, not least of which was my afterschool-special kind of upbringing, that I should have a baby. I concluded that since I probably shouldn't breed with such a wayward set of data points, I didn't want to. Either way, it just wasn't the best idea for me, this whole baby business. It was a can of worms I didn't want to open, particularly for someone who didn't even own a decent can opener.

But then those sperm did something surprisingly smart, if indifferent to my wishes. They pulled out all the stops. They brought their best men. They got up there when the getting was still good. They got past the rigorous background checks and carnivalesque feats of strength and fired off a winner.

And I took one look at that plus sign, exhaled the last cloud of cigarette smoke I would ever taste, and said, "Fuuuuuuuuck."

. . .

The moral of my story? If I can go from a cat- and smoke-filled Krystals trailer sort of life to raising a happy, darling, healthy baby, then the sky is the literal limit for literally anyone who literally even sort of tries. Literally.

But I won't lie to you: What you're about to face is a strange, unprecedented journey into feelings, weight gain, farts, ear zits, judgment, confusion, hilarity, terror, and the sense that something small but motivated is putting a lot of pressure on your bladder. You might also be extremely horny. (Normally, being judged a lot isn't a turn-on for most people, but you never know.)

What counts here is that every day, in every way, women just like you and me find ourselves in this very drawers-dropped-in-a-field predicament. Sometimes it's out of nowhere, like in that show *I Didn't Know I Was Pregnant*, where women don't know they are pregnant until their babies literally crawl up their chests and start breastfeeding.

But that's not you. Thank God, that's not you. You've done something right, here—you already know you're pregnant right now. So, congrats!

If we can have our druthers, nothing will be crawling out of you into the toilet. See? In spite of how shocked you might feel, you have not, in fact, been sucker-punched by this news after all. At least not literally.

Sure, it's terrifying in both the horror-movie and existential-fear sense, whether this is your first baby or your fifth. But that would be true whether you read any books or thought about crib sheets or not—having a baby is a hella big deal regardless of how many lists you can make in advance. And since you've decided to do this, the important thing to remember is that you can do this. You really can. Because I did it.

Know this: Even as motherhood feels like it's hurtling at you through space with almost no time to prep, you actually *do* have all the time you need to get it together. Also, "mother" may feel like the only "you" there is now, but it is merely one designation among the many monikers of your life. It alone does not define you. Even if it's covered in clichés about mashed yams, stepping up to the plate, doing it and taking responsibility, and being a whole person and all that crap.

Welcome to motherhood. First shot of apple cider vinegar is on me.

2.

DID I SCREW UP MY CHANCES FOR A HEALTHY BABY?

When you have no plans to grow a baby, what then, pray tell, is to prevent you from eating a bunch of mercury-coated raw fish, dropping to the floor in an amateur belly flop to do the snake, or taking matador classes? Nothing, that's what.

Given your carefree lifestyle, you were likely engaged in any number of the following activities prior to The Big Bang: drinking, smoking, bouncing, air-traffic controlling, eating excessive amounts of tuna and deli meat, drinking unpasteurized milk, having an ill-advised summer of coke, listening to Maroon 5, reading *Fifty Shades of Grey*, catching bowling balls right in the gut, or merely getting really, really into *Here Comes Honey Boo Boo*. All wildly fun things; all terrible for an unborn child.

Your first response to the news of this pregnancy is likely to be, like mine, an unforgettable "how the hell did this happen?!" moment. Your second thought is likely to be: "Shit, did I fuck up my baby?" Short answer: Maybe? Technically-just-as-short-but-long answer that's likely more correct: Probably not? It's hard to say, but at least the ambiguity of this question will prepare you well for parenting, when there is literally no one right answer to any question. Every topic can be and is contradicted and debated with gusto and verve.

Not only was I sure I'd fucked up my baby, but I was more sure that I would be prosecuted in a court of judgment the moment I waltzed into my obstetrician's office to confirm this surprise pregnancy. He would see my sallow skin, depressed posture, and immature attitude and immediately pen a brilliant article for a reputable medical journal titled "Can She Be Real (or Helped)? The Most Horribly Irresponsible Pregnant Woman I've Ever Encountered."

I was about as ready to face that chorus of medical judgment as I was ready to change a diaper, so I tossed the beer, dropped the cigarette into the pregnant-positive pee-filled toilet for one last satisfying singe, and turned immediately to the wilderness of the Internet to find out exactly how horribly I had damaged my progeny.

Drinking? Check. Smoking? Check. Willfully depriving my body of useful nutrition and/or decent amounts of sunlight and water? Check. Bouncing up and down idiotically on a jet ski? Check.

But what I found was oddly reassuring: If nothing else, it was at least a very popular Google search. About a bajillion other reckless boozehounds just like me had searched the exact same thing, and damn near every variation on this question, which boils down to: "I was drinking/smoking/getting high/using drugs/being an idiot before I knew I was pregnant. Is my baby okay?"

Let me just interject here that I'm sure we can all agree that the Internet is full of outliers who are drawn to its anonymity and conflicting information—information from which you may easily cherry-pick the most reassuring of outcomes for yourself and call it a bloated day. None of it replaces that thing you really do have to do, reader: go to an actual doctor who will actually tell you to your face how horrible you actually were/are. Studies on pregnant women and the effects of bad things on their unborn children are notoriously hard to conduct, since no sane person wants to coke it up while pregnant for the sake of science. Furthermore, the results of these types of studies are mixed even when they are available, which is why no obstetrician can guarantee that your pregnancy is going to be smooth sailing no matter what you've partaken in prior to or just after conceiving.

But until your caregiver tells you things are looking A-OK, think of using the Internet as a kind of great practice for being looked at, judged, and given unsolicited advice in real life. FYI, being judged and given unsolicited advice is about to be a daily occurrence for the rest of your pregnancy and child-rearing life, so open arms, people. Open arms.

But back to the very closed arms of the digital safety net: There's a kind of truth in this outlier mob madness. That is to say, a bajillion other people searched just as you did, having committed egregious pre-pregnant crimes eerily similar to yours, and yet SOMEHOW the horror stories, the tales of damage and woe, are not as ever-present as you might think.

"In case you didn't know, pregnant women are notorious for Googling scary crap about their pregnancies."

—Christine Gilbert

These people were just like you with their *Risky Business*–level bad behavior, and they reported that their babies turned out just fine. Better than fine! Great, even! I sighed with what had to be at least a double pregnant pause, comforted by the knowledge that I had probably as good a chance as anyone—or at least our grandparents' generation—of having a healthy pregnancy. I would save the emotional question for the next nine lifetimes.

But you won't get off that easy, friend. What you will find out there may be temporarily reassuring, but it isn't a guarantee of anything and still comes with a finger wag. The online anecdotes run the gamut, from "ARE YOU STUPID? Every single thing you drink or eat directly impacts your baby's SAT scores!" to "Dude, chill. I smoked five joints a day, and my baby is hella cool." That's because for practically every single study out there about what's good or bad for you during pregnancy, there seems to be an equally convincing study that found just the opposite. Whether you're smoking, drinking, taking folic acid, or dyeing your hair—or not doing that stuff—gestation is a gamble, no matter how you slice it.

In between these extremes of "do it" and "oh shit, don't do it," lies the also-hella-cool concept of pragmatism. She's your new best friend, even though you ignored her when you thought it was a good idea to shoot Grand Marnier or not contribute to a 401(k). Practically speaking, says our friend, it seems like there would have to be some kind of basic biological protection for a growing fetus in the early stages in the womb, a Hail Mary for the initial Big Bang, a protective cloak for nature's little bean sprout to take hold without fear of every errant wind uprooting her. Right? How else could so many of us have unplanned pregnancies and mostly turn out okay (debatable!)?

I will leave the medical science to an actual doctor who has written outrageously successful journal articles. But consider my theory that for the first few weeks of pregnancy—during the time you don't even know you are pregnant and wouldn't even test positive on a prego piss test—perhaps there is a kind of safe passage from the land of the partying to the land of the sober. Again, don't take my word for it; the evidence for this is mixed. The guarantees of a healthy pregnancy—whether you do all the "right" things or not—are zero. But still. Isn't it possible that it is possible, given how many of us are having these things by accident?

When I waltzed into that doctor's office, I told that graying Stanley Tucci look-alike of mine everything: the drinking, the drugs, the burritos, the lack of sunlight. It all came tumbling out like the effects of one too many happy hour two-for-ones on an empty stomach. He smirked, gave me and the husband a quick once-over, and told me not to worry, no-nonsense style. To just stop what I had been doing and hit the straight and narrow. And, of course, he said to hold off on announcing the pregnancy until I was past twelve weeks—not because I was a boozehound smoker who may as well have been catching bowling balls in the gut for a living, but because I was OLD (ahem, thirty-three at the time of conception).

My experience, again, is not to be substituted for your own medical provider giving you the classic lecture of ambiguous reassurance. I offer my story here only to say that either I had the world's most cavalier doctor, or there is something to this incubational-free-pass-early-on-for-expecting-mothers theory, even the unexpecting kind, whose bodies need a bit of time to prepare for the long haul ahead.

Whoever or whatever out there did that for us and our bodies? Thanks. We totes owe ya one. Luckily, I hadn't taken Accutane for a decade, and my hard-drug days were long gone. It was "only" the smoking and drinking I'd had to quit.

But rest assured that as long as your caregiver is not worried, then you needn't be, either. So while your baby is kickin' it, you can kick it, too. Just not how you used to. Remember how you used to? That was fun? Buh-bye.

I don't mean to be cavalier about the mountain-moving levels of willpower you will have to muster to drop whatever bad habits you may have recklessly pursued for the duration of this pregnancy thus far. I cannot to this day fully explain how I was able to rally the troops myself. I only knew that, for me, continuing to smoke was not an option. I just couldn't do it. And I didn't really feel like smoking anyway. That's what is so great about the discomfort of early pregnancy, if you can call it "great" to feel like your insides are mobilizing to be your outsides. When everything is ripe for the hurling up, the last thing you want to do is add toxic chemicals to the mix. Like the thought of alcohol the morning after with a wincing hangover, most of the time, your old vices won't even be a thing to fight. The rest of the time, you will be a fierce warrior against vice.

That said, as anyone who's ever tried a mood-altering substance can tell you: there's always a poor man's substitute. You'll be shocked and pleasantly surprised to learn that once all vices have been thoroughly eliminated from your bloodstream, you've basically reset yourself to what other people consider normal operating levels. This means that regular, old, over-the-counter, widely available, safe-during-pregnancy medicinals and natural highs can now give you that classic take-the-edge-off feeling you once turned to booze and smokes for. For instance:

» When I needed a pick-me-up, one tall Starbucks coffee had me pretty much bouncing off the walls. And my child. (One cup of coffee a day is perfectly safe during pregnancy, says the American Pregnancy Association, which recommends keeping daily intake to a moderate 150 to 300 mg.)

» If you're not the coffee-drinking type, there's always a little piece of dark chocolate, or a cup of black tea.

» Here are a few other things you might want to do for a mood shifter when the going gets really safe, healthy, and boring:
  - *Sex*
  - *Baths*
  - *Showers*
  - *Walks*
  - *A glass of wine*
  - *One Excedrin*
  - *Two ibuprofen and a cup of coffee ("poor, pregnant woman's speedball")*

Just think, eventually you'll have a child and it will be just as difficult to find time to have a beer or two, but at least then you won't feel guilty about it. (Unless you're breastfeeding.)

But until then, now that you know that you got away with something, feel free to use the knowledge of this free pass both ways:

1. To rationalize any bad behavior prior to knowing you were pregnant

2. To now become one of those unbearable, overly concerned pregnant women who can't even walk through a cloud of Lysol spray for fear of the harm it will do to her child

Sure, it's a huge, flip-floppy contradiction, but no one expects a pregnant woman to make sense. Sheesh, it's not like you're running for political office. (I really hope you are not running for political office, because then I cannot help you at all.)

3.

ARE THERE ANY DISADVANTAGES TO AN UNPLANNED PREGNANCY?

As the wise, sadly anonymous person on "Yahoo Answers" said succinctly in response to the question, "What are the disadvantages to unplanned pregnancy?":

"Only one: You're pregnant."

4.

TEN ADVANTAGES TO AN UNPLANNED PREGNANCY

Granted, "Surprise Pregnancy at Thirty-Five" is on approximately no one's bucket list, but this caution-to-the-wind adventure nonetheless offers a surprising number of advantages you might not expect from anything so terrifying. To wit:

1. You'll Get Healthier, Faster

Sure, you were going to do a cleanse and start that new workout routine on Monday. Of next year. If nothing else, this pregnancy is the final uterine push you needed to cut out the fried, salty foods in tiny individually wrapped packages that you're so obsessed with; focus on healthier stress management techniques that don't involve your ex-boyfriend, craft beers, and 3:00 A.M.; and start eating something—anything—resembling a green vegetable. And no, I'm not talking about those snap pea crisps.

2. You'll Get Emotionally Sorted Out

With the right outfit, being a basket case in your twenties was precious. Unforch, no maternity outfit in the world makes being a *pregnant* basket case look cute. Luckily, pregnancy puts a natural, and surprisingly manageable, deadline on getting your shit together upstairs, at least enough to focus completely on another human being.

That's good news, because your feelings about your mother, your life, and every relationship you may have ever contemplated might come rushing up faster than a bad case of heartburn after some buffalo wings. Will you actually resolve all your complicated baggage before the birth? Of course not. All the more reason to start chipping away at the heap of hassle in your life now. And seriously—put your back into it. Also, don't forget to pair those wings with some (organic) ranch dressing.

3. You Have an Ironclad Excuse to Get Out of Things

Most people wouldn't characterize pregnancy as convenient. It may be a tumultuous time of medically unexplainable sensations, sure, but it's also your get-out-of-jail-free card for any person or thing you don't feel like seeing/doing for the next nine months, give or take five years. This is great news for anyone who's just been guilted into joining the company softball team, or anyone who has a really hard time saying no to trivia night. If you already have kids, you're probably familiar with this excuse. It's even *stronger* now that you're pregnant again!

But even better, it's a legit reason to stop doing a bunch of bad stuff you always meant to quit and now actually can't do in good conscience anymore, as we discussed a couple of chapters ago.

4. You'll Simplify Your Life

You think pregnancy just made your life infinitely more complicated, but looked at from another angle, it just became ridiculously clear what matters. Hint: Not the weekend in the mountains where you will watch your twelve closest friends engage in a competitive drunk farting match. Remember all that stuff you needed to do to become a real grown-up but were putting off because it seemed confusing or impossible? You know, like building up a real savings account, creating a will, or getting a life insurance policy. Before your every waking moment is allocated to properly sanitizing bottles, deal with that kind of shit now.

5. You'll Figure Out Your Career

Babies kill more than slim thighs—if your job is going out all night, every night, wining and dining clients and being available at a moment's notice, your career could be the next to go. But a baby can also bring into sharp focus what was otherwise blurry: your net worth, your career options, and your real ambitions.

If you're lucky enough to have a good salary, this could mean taking steps to hire or share a nanny to help when you're at work. Or maybe you're not that happy with your job anyway, and it's time to think about going back to school in the short term to get the training you need to start a new career. (Yes, it seems insane to enroll in a class while pregnant. Now picture doing it with an infant. Suddenly pregnant schooling seems totally manageable.) Alternately, you might want to find a way to take some time off, either as a few-month maternity leave or something more long-term.

Whatever you choose to do, it will never be clearer what you really want to do with your life. This baby is not an impediment so much as a very squirmy piece of the puzzle.

Getting pregnant made one thing crystal clear for me: Hanging out in the club getting older while everyone else stayed twenty-four was no way for a lady to live out her twilight years; plus, babies can't do shots. I was already burned out from hitting shows and living at bars, but this was my official, unquestionable excuse to jump while I could. And jump I did. My baby was my gold-plated parachute. You might find that this pregnancy puts your future into focus, too.

6. You'll Finally Clean Your House

Literally. Hey, maybe you were already a really organized neat freak, in which case this pregnancy must really be throwing you for a loop. But if you're more like the rest of us, you probably never did spring cleaning in the first place, aren't technically sure what a duvet cover is, and wouldn't know how to degrease an oven if it came with a magic wand.

Luckily, you have nine very long months to get your house in order. Yes, looong. It seems like you have to do everything right now, and you do, but trust me, in retrospect it will seem like these months were the last slow-paced, lackadaisical vacation of your life. If it's not your first, you can finally get around to donating some of those old toys and clothes to make space for this new bundle of thing-accumulating joy.

For me, getting my house in order meant cleaning up an ungodly amount of cat hair and cat crap. It meant desmokifying a house that I don't think had ever seen twenty-four hours straight of fresh air in the four years I'd lived there. I also had to kick out some roommates. It meant making a space outside of my uterus to welcome a baby, in a home that I could actually be proud of. Which was more than I'd ever been able to say about my uterus, or my closets. Whatever issues you have in *your* home, this is a good opportunity to overcome them.

7. You'll Figure Out Your Finances

You would not believe how much money you can save—even when you work as a reporter at a tiny little alt-weekly in the South that you know for sure is underpaying you based on the national average, common sense, your eyes, gossip, and your paycheck. When you stop drinking, smoking, buying large coffees, and eating lunch and dinner out every day, you can live on practically nothing in some towns.

If you already have kids, will this one tip the scale financially—as in, will the cost of daycare outpace your income if you work outside the home? Should you consider options beyond what you currently do?

Yes, sacrifice is hard, but regret is a bitter mistress. It would have been really hard to brag about how much I had my shit together if my kid had to pay for her own car seat.

8. You'll Figure Out Your Relationship

Nothing says "Are we gonna last?" like making things real permanent with a museum-quality reproduction of you and your significant other. I won't mince words: Having a baby on the fly can fuck your shit up faster than a failed Breathalyzer. This is where you have to get really Zen, and get out of your own head, and get really big picture about your sitch. It's helpful to think of this as the ultimate test, because it pretty much is. You want to take this journey with someone who understands as well as you do—which is not at all yet, but with an openness to the full extent of the word—what sacrifice is going to be required.

The good news is that having a big crazy talk with yourself and your baby daddy will definitely clear a few things up. The bad news is, you may wish things had stayed foggy. But now is not the time for uncertainty. You need hard facts, firm commitments, and a partner who is ready to pull an American-hero moment with you.

But not everyone takes to big platitudes. If having a kid together on the fly screws up the relationship, you must consider it a sad but positive lesson learned early. If it makes your relationship stronger— which is not unheard of—you've just scored yourself the unicorn of happiness, a double rainbow of a blessing. Google it. I dare you.

9. You'll Embrace a Roll-with-It Kinda Attitude

If you are the anxious, planning type, having a baby on the fly is proof positive that things that pop up (or out, as the case may be) unexpectedly are sometimes life's best lessons. I know, it's so cheesy, and yet it is so true. Perhaps you can't see it now or can only sense its presence just off in the distance, but getting your shit together at a moment's notice for your hilarious and awesome child will no doubt remain among the top best things you ever did. If you already have a kid(s), wait till you see them with their new sibling. The magic is hard to argue with.

But if right now all this just sounds like a bunch of pep-talky silver linings in a cloud of stormy weather, take comfort from the drizzle with some science: In 1999, researchers in the stormy weather capital of Glasgow, Scotland, found that, contrary to all conventional wisdom ever, rolling with it has tangible benefits! The study, published in the *British Journal of Medical Psychology*, showed that unexpectedly pregnant ladies who rolled with life's tiny little kicks and punches had vastly greater scores for "cementing relationships with their partner, family and friends, of improving their work and social life, and even of getting better housing."

Which leads me to another advantage of unexpected gestation . . .

10. You'll Get All Focused

There's nothing like pregnancy to make you latch on to every last resource you've got like it's sliding off a cliff, or dive over that cliff in search of better ones. Your mind, though strangely foggy and muddled, will also become preternaturally attuned to free time, opportunities, and efficiency-minded solutions. What was once a blur of gotta-get-around-to will become a clear-eyed to-do list, and the weird thing is, for what might be the first time in your life, you will actually find yourself getting it done.

5.

WILL MY LIFE BE OVER?

Do you ever get the feeling, while you're sitting around at home feeling lumpy and gestational, that everyone has rented a lovably rustic cabin together in the mountains to do 'shrooms without you? Congratulations, you're that unique kind of pregnant where you are both paranoid and totally correct at the same time. Enjoy it. It doesn't come around often in this lifetime.

What's more, you're not even sure if you care. Of course you care somewhere in the dark, dusty prolactin-riddled corners of your hormone-jacked brain, but do you care enough to do anything about it? Oh, look: jalapeño hot wings.

Where were we? Right. Can you still get your old-time kicks when the only thing kicking is a fetus inside you? Depends. Some pregnant women are industrious uberschnitzels who can still do it all, managing to maintain a full social calendar and a discernible waist. They actually stand up, go to social events, shop, host dinners, and hit parties while abstaining from alcohol and deli meat. Others (ahem, ME) are tired, schlumpy, and long-suffering, and will only be found performing tasks that are legally required to keep a job, any other children they have, and on occasion, a husband.

Add to that the unique emotional ass-weight of not having been ready to embark on this motherhood journey right now (or at all), and you might find yourself like I did, stuck somewhere in the middle, struggling to maintain some semblance of my old life while at least having the good sense to stop mainlining burritos and Yuenglings.

It wasn't easy. You can be ready to take your life in a new direction but unsure how, exactly, to leave the old one behind. But everyone's situation is different. If you're a grad student studying early-childhood education while working three days a week at a daycare, I'd say you're a helluva lot more prepared to venture into motherhood-on-fast-forward than someone who rarely wakes up before 9:00 A.M. and breakfasts on a bag of old french fries you found under your car seat. Or maybe you have one lovely child and are relishing your life as a manageable party of three. Regardless, you may find yourself straddling your former and future lives while you live in your current pregnant state.

Here's how I handled it. At first, I hung out with friends, showed up for post-work drinks and sipped water, and tried to maintain an interest in social goings-on. This worked for approximately one week. Then I quickly discovered that without the social lubricant of booze, it turned out that people I once thought were interesting actually only talked about television and weed. When subjects came up that I would have normally suffered through on a good buzz, or worse, enjoyed, I now felt bored and annoyed. Who were these gargoyles that never talked about ideas or current events? Was I actually just standing around making fun of everyone in my head while slightly drunk for the last fifteen years?

What's more, now that I couldn't even crack a good joke during this completely sober regime, I was suddenly No Longer Fun to my social group. Not that I'd realized this quite yet. Sure, I could get them to join me for Monday lunches at Cracker Barrel, but it took a rude awakening to realize it wasn't my company they came for but the biscuits. I was blindsided by this lesson in the form of a convo with a bunch of drunken, seafaring adventurers I used to call friends.

Friend #1 to Friend #2 while I'm sitting RIGHT THERE: "You know what would be so cool? Adventuring in Japan!"

Friend #2 to Friend #1 while I'm sitting RIGHT THERE: "JAPAN!?!? Shall we call it Adventure Number Four for this summer?" (Note: This summer. When I would be navigating life with a newborn.)

I know what you're thinking and, yes, it's totally okay to hate them for already having three other adventures lined up that they didn't even tell me about—you don't even have to be pregnant to hate that. Secondly, everyone laughed and agreed that they would all "adventure" together. Thirdly, yes, they used "adventure" as a verb. People, apparently, are doing this now.

Fourthly, you and I both know they will never go to Japan together—that requires actual planning while not drunk and a bunch of disposable income. Fifth, what is actually bothersome here is not Japan, and not plans, and not people going to Japan without you. It is accepting in that everyday way that, for the foreseeable future, you can no longer even pretend that you can drop everything and go to the mall, much less Japan. And sixth: summers!? Since when are summers still a carefree time you have off to plan fun things anyway, as if you're just fresh out of college?

But most importantly, no one looked my way with so much as an obligatory, pitying invitational glance about Japan. I was a DOA travel friend as far as they were concerned. Technically, I was worse than DOA; I was whatever comes before DOA. Dead. It's just called dead.

Prior to the Japan discussion, I would say I was more than satisfied with my decision to breed. Sure, I had made the decision once the breeding was well under way, but I meant it, and I'd partied more than enough. Friday night at home seemed oddly attractive after years of going out four nights a week or more.

So what, fellow pregos, was this particular feeling coming over me? Annoyance? Gas? Irritation? Oh, no. Actual, honest-to-god jealousy. Here I was, happily standing in my truth—okay, sitting, always sitting—and without the slightest warning or provocation, along came the chugging train of holy-shit-here's-something-you-didn't-even-realize-you-wanted-to-do-but-now-you-can't.

I give you this example merely to illustrate that even the most resilient choice-choosers among us are still going to have moments of verklempty doubt about our decision to abandon the ship of carefree spontaneity for that changing table on dry land. You were perfectly fine just waddling through your life committed to your decision, yesiree, when suddenly you got a pang of something that stopped you dead in your tracks.

Moreover, if you don't have friends, travel plans, or a social life anymore now that you're in your isolation booth of pregnancy, what's left? What kind of life is this, anyway?

Um, got a Netflix subscription still? Hulu? Hope you're a reader. Any hobbies? Because that's going to make this a lot easier.

"The first half of our life is ruined by our parents and the second half by our children."

—Clarence Darrow

It's worth noting that even though going to Japan sounds mighty fun, it's not really about Japan, or a last-minute weekend road trip to the mountains, or reading the Sunday paper while smoking cigarettes uninterrupted so you can linger just-so on a good sentence, take a drag, exhale, and re-read. It's just good, old-fashioned pregnancy cold feet. I realize that there is no single solitary part of your body during pregnancy that ever seems to feel actually cold, but stick with me here.

It's that nagging feeling that everyone you know is out together right now enjoying some kind of young, life-defining spontaneity while you're incubating in a deep couch imprint. It's that maybe you ditched on a road you weren't ready to get off of just yet. It's that maybe you hadn't quite finished up with all the carefree, responsibility-averse living, or that perhaps, God help you, you were never going to be finished.

It's times like these when it would be really, really helpful for you to witness a conversation between Current You and Future You, *It's a Wonderful Life*–style, so you could see what you didn't know yet already. You would learn that you will be totally fine—and not just fine but better, even. For me, that conversation would have gone something like this:

Future Me: "Look, remember *Sliding Doors*? You're Gwyneth Paltrow at the subway right now, and you could waltz right into that subway car or accidentally trip on something going down the stairs, which will slow you down and make you miss that subway car, which means your husband is cheating on you? Wait, this isn't coming out right."

Current Me: "Sigh. Does this story end with the cool, blonde haircut or the mousy brown one?"

Future Me: "Duh—the cool one? I mean, at first, it's the mousy brown one. But then you get sick of that and you get the cool blonde one. It's going to crack open your entire life and just bombard it with all kinds of light."

Current Me: "Light bombardment? That's what I'm going for? Does this light bombardment come with a smoking section?"

Future Me: "Right, I forgot! Burned-out, crusty rock chick/barfly was such a solid life plan. What was your exit strategy again?"

Current Me: "This better be one hell of a kid."

Future Me: "It is! It has your sense of humor! And mannerisms! And your husband's science brain! It is pure, uncorrupted love! It will elevate your entire existence! It blows all that other shit out of the water!"

Current Me: "Even Japan? Even sleeping late? Even cigarettes?"

Future Me: "Gah, you're asking the wrong questions."

Current Me: "What's the right question?"

Future Me: "Is it worth it?"

Current Me: "Okay, is it worth it?"

Future Me: "If you knew how much, you'd have done it ten years ago."

6.

BUT I'M NOT EVEN A BABY PERSON!

In spite of what our ~~deepest wishes~~ celebrity tabloids tell us, a baby is not, in fact, an accessory. But that doesn't mean this child's unexpected arrival won't a) drastically alter your wardrobe and b) cause an existential crisis on par with what happened that time you took that quiz that instructed you to "find your season." To wit: the stark realization that you are not, never were, and are never gonna be a baby person. Only now you're going to have a baby.

A baby person, of course, is someone who appears so suited to the carrying and care of children, so naturally maternal, so effortlessly comforting—see: my mother-in-law—that when your brain tries to conjure them without childr—nope, it can't do it.

They live and breathe children, look natural dancing gaily around in flower-filled fields, and are forever threatening to morph into Mary Poppins. What's more, they actually *like* babies, what with their near-constant cries, blobby necks, and built-to-be-agitating pitch, not to mention their batshit preference to be with you every single second of their budding lives. I know, right? Insane.

Then there are the rest of us: nonbaby people who don't even know what to say to the little bugger, who couldn't hold a baby's head upright if our lives depended on it. And like a person without a hat head being given a hat, or a non-watch-arm-haver being asked to put on a watch, a nonbaby person with a baby is an awkward sight to behold. It just doesn't go together.

It's not your fault, per se. We can't all be baby people. Some of us have actually managed to carve out lives where we were never around children. Some of us can plainly see with our own child-free eyes that babies are, in fact, weird, terrifying, disease-carrying, nonsensical creatures who follow no rhyme or reason. Some of us took one look at *The Exorcist* and realized immediately what it really was: a metaphor for toddlerhood.

Maybe it's just that babies don't do anything for you, or you don't know how to act around them, or their lack of conversation skills leaves you in a perpetual state of awkward enthusiasm, and all you can think about is exactly how many seconds can pass before you can hand this thing back to its mother without being accused of lacking a soul?

That was me. If I could not muster the appropriate enthusiasm for other people's children, how would I ever do it for my own? What's more, my very fast-paced, bar-loving, outgoing existence and life in the blogosphere depended entirely on sarcasm and detachment, the opposite of baby person-ness. I wouldn't have known an uninhibited compassionate impulse or a goofy game of peekaboo if it toddled right up to me and offered a hug. Hugs—gross.

But I would need more than just compassionate impulses to navigate the newborn obstacle course. There are also all those games you play with babies, a whole world out there in need of narrating in a fun, upbeat voice, and an untold number of life-affirming facial expressions I'd need to soothe this new person in my life. And that was just the stuff I could remember seeing moms do in diaper commercials.

Furthermore, what about other easy-for-a-baby-person activities I might also suck at, like making appropriately silly faces? I'd also have to say "good job" a lot, and say it convincingly when the "job" was something like rolling from tummy to back.

I was sure I couldn't hack it. For instance, it once took me two whole weeks to love a kitten I'd adopted, whereas my noncommittal, totally-willing-to-mooch ex-boyfriend loved it at first sight. If a scruffy bum could muster instant love for something he wasn't even related to, how long would it take me to love my own child?

I was in big trouble. But I also wasn't alone. Google "not a baby person" and you'll see that plenty of women are just as mortified as you are, wondering if their inability to go ga-ga over other people's pods means they'll come up wanting with their own.

One woman confessed on a forum that she just didn't "get" babies. Another said she couldn't have been bothered with them. But story after story of baby-love blind spots were followed up with the only one thing that can assure you: that when their baby wheeled into their lives, all the right stuff kicked in. Whew. (Babies are on wheels?)

If baby things and baby feelings—comforting a tiny living thing or conjuring marathon-levels of enthusiasm when you are not the mad-enthusiasm type (and have no access to Lance Armstrong–levels of doping drugs)—sound utterly terrifying to you, too, rest assured your baby grades on a very generous curve. As long as you are loving, and as long as you are there.

Believe me, the nurturing will come. The enthusiasm will come. Eventually, you will startle at the stranger you hear using what sounds like a naturally gushing tone when cooing at your baby, even when reading the words of some of the more offensively saccharine kids' books out there, and realize that the stranger is you. And you won't even totally hate this new person, no matter how uncool she looks now.

And if the naturally up-with-people vibe never hits at your corner of the universe, something more important is happening anyway. Unless you took some really weird drugs, your baby won't be a baby forever. That's right, just when you get this whole infant thing hammered out, you'll wake up one day and realize that your baby's blobby neck is a normal neck, her blobby legs are standing, wobbly legs. And what you may discover is that for every way that you were not a baby person, you are in fact, a toddler person. You might even be really, really good at it.

HELP!...
HOW TO DEAL WITH PREGNANCY OBSTACLES

7.

WHAT WILL PEOPLE SAY ABOUT ME?
(Because I Know They Will Say Things)

Try as you might to hide your pregnancy with ferns and baggy clothes, it will eventually get out that you're with child (plus, there's always a preternatural pregnancy sniffer in your office who can tell immediately—and she is a huge gossip). If you're lucky, this news will be welcomed with nothing but positivity, well-wishing, and good vibes. If it was at all obvious that you were not suited to mother anything, the news might be met with a little cognitive dissonance. There are typically four possible reactions you're going to get when word of your surprise pregnancy gets out.

The Well-Wishers
These are people who either don't know, don't care, or simply are more evolved about how pregnancy works. Maybe they are religious and view all pregnancies as God's blessings. Maybe they are just sweet, good-hearted people who like babies and children and treat their impending arrival as a wonderful thing worth celebrating. They have basic good faith that you're going to be a great mother who will pull it all together and do this thing right.

Things They Say: "Congratulations!" "So wonderful!" "How can I help?"

How to Handle: With genuine kindness and appreciation. Even if they end up being too into your pregnancy, or wanting to relive their own vicariously, or very weirdly religious and want you to be, too, they are an invaluable resource for talking endlessly about yourself or just wanting to feel super stoked. Plus, having people so excited about this crazy, madcap thing you're going to do has a way of easing the discomfort.

The Dicks

Maybe they are unrefined, maybe they are assholes, but these people immediately sensed your pregnancy was not on purpose, and they will let you know immediately with irritating tones and faux concern.

Things They Say: "Surprise! Congrats?" "Really??" "Are you HAPPY?"

How to Handle: Ignore. If you must, say something in response like "Gee, I guess I know who not to invite to the baby shower." But it's helpful to understand the background of a response like this. Obviously, there's still a lingering taboo about a surprise baby, as if accidents can't be happy, as if unplanned always means unwanted. For most of the history of the universe, surprise pregnancies have been viewed with embarrassment, taboo, or suspicion—you know, when women weren't being shipped off to have their babies in secret to avoid the family-ruining shame.

Pregnancy and childrearing are wonderful but terrifying, blissful but exhausting, miraculous but mundane—and that's when you do it on purpose. When it's by accident, it's still all that stuff, too, only you just might need a minute to catch up with the shock. So does society. Try to have patience with the dicks whose hearts and minds are so dick-like that they cannot see the happy in this accident.

The Silent Judgies

No one is saying rude things to your face; they just aren't saying anything at all. This can be even more annoying and anxiety-inducing, especially if it means friends, coworkers, and family are less inclined to shower you with well-wishing because they aren't sure you're happy about it. While this makes some kind of sense, it can have the unfortunate side effect of making you feel like your pregnancy is the elephant in the room. You know, the same room you're sitting in, feeling like an actual elephant?

Things They Say:

How to Handle: There's not much you can say to people who aren't saying anything to your face. But you might be able to imagine why they are unsure how to react: Maybe you inadvertently made your pregnancy really juicy gossip by being very public about your aversion to breeding, such as I was when I actually wrote about how I would never breed (uh, never say never?). Maybe you seem openly thrown by the news. Maybe you seem happy, but that happiness seems tenuous. Maybe you seem totally batshit—and who would blame you?

Try not to imagine what they are saying behind your back, unless you are privy to a direct source in the form of a rat. I was told that people were saying awful, hilarious things about my pregnancy, such as: *OMG! Did you hear? A vowed nonbreeder is breeding! What happened? Maybe she's old? Maybe she's desperate? I heard she has a weird uterus! Can you imagine HER as a mother?*

I also happened to be in a social scene filled with hyenas who were more resistant to growing up than even I was. It was enough to make me wish I'd hidden it up until the very last moment, staging a water-balloon fight to cover my water breaking.

You, however, probably hang around with people who are slightly more mature. If so, try projecting your acceptance of this situation. Try making a well-placed joke, or an honest acknowledgement that you had no plans to have kids, but now that you're pregnant, you're going for it. Who can say anything rude to that?

The Nosy People

If we're talking about nosy friends, that's one thing. If it's some rando working the mailroom who you don't even talk to, it's a bit disconcerting.

What They Say: "Wow, so did you *want* to be pregnant?"

How to Handle: Since slapping them with your steamed prosciutto is not an option, I say respond with, "I don't know, did you mean to sound like a prying wildebeest?" If that's too harsh, tap into your newfound patience as a soon-to-be mother and channel your best Kate Moss via Johnny Depp: "Never complain; never explain." Give them nothing to feed their silent judgment that you can't even be sure exists because they are so silent, but fuck, you're hormonal as hell, which makes you feel oddly intuitive.

Of course, Johnny Depp was giving advice to Moss about being famous, but this advice actually works rather excellently for us, because an unplanned pregnancy can make you a temporary celebrity in your town, office, or social circle. We sure do love when someone is caught off-guard in direct contradiction with their stated goals, and we love to see if the wear and tear will show on them. Expect to be looked at, analyzed, and gossiped about, even as people wish you well. Just never complain; never explain. Never complain; never explain. It has a nice ring to it.

But if that sounds like utter bullshit, and you don't feel like acting the part of the stoically together pregnant woman, I salute you. Consider actually educating these poor souls who don't know how mean they sound or how disappointing their responses can be.

Start by introducing your bafflingly ignorant colleagues to this phrase: *unplanned but not unwanted.*

Try practicing it out loud, alone, and then later, with a partner. Make sure you say it cheerfully. Think chirpy, endlessly patient, and somewhat pitying. It might help to pretend you are Snow White or Glinda the Good Witch when you say it, because this can help conjure the correct tone and posture you want: that of a very privileged, special, extraordinarily more evolved person having to explain to an unfortunate, hyena-faced plebe that you do in fact want the baby you have chosen to have. Because, you know, if you didn't want it? You WOULDN'T HAVE IT.

Explaining "Unplanned but Not Unwanted"

Real talk: The concept of an unplanned pregnancy is still full of stereotypes, but especially one big one: that all unplanned pregnancies are unwanted. There are studies we needn't cite about the lack of resources given to "unplanned" children. While I am perfectly willing to concede that many unplanned pregnancies ARE, in fact, unwanted and result in loads of unpleasant circumstances that will break your heart, we should never assume that the phrase "happy accident" is always some kind of generous but sad euphemism.

Sometimes we find ourselves staring down a new path we hadn't even seen the first time we whizzed by it, and we never regret taking it. It really is both happy and an accident. The mind reels, I know. It might not be the Norman Rockwell painting of pregnancies, but nothing is.

If you feel like it—and believe me, something about pregnancy hormones makes you want to tear into anyone who dares to tell you how to feel about anything—consider trying out this monologue if ever confronted in an inappropriate way about your particular situation:

Ahem. There are lots of kinds of unplanned pregnancies, concerned citizen. There is, unfortunately, unplanned and unwanted, the one you seem so familiar with: "Oh, look, honey. Here is another unwanted hemorrhoid I never expected growing out of MY ASS."

Then there is planned and unwanted: "Oh no, I ordered this lifetime supply of blue cheese. I thought I would enjoy it for my entire life and here I am one week in and so, so sick of blue cheese. Whatever shall I do?"

And then there is planned and wanted: "I love the dick out of blueberries, so I'm going to get some blueberries, and then I am going to eat them. Damn, these blueberries are everything I imagined them to be. I love blueberries."

But then there is the magical Goldilocks of unexpected pregnancies: unplanned but wanted. As in, "Oh, I didn't PLAN on seeing Moonrise Kingdom *tonight, honey, but look, you went and surprised me by ordering it. I'd never even heard of it, but it turns out I think it's an awesome movie!"*

What I am saying here, my nosy little mouth-breather, is that my baby is like Moonrise Kingdom. *I might not have ever gotten around to seeing it had I not accidently found it playing on iTunes, but I'm sure glad I did. It's a terrific film. I'll love it forever. My, what a sight to behold it is. I sure hope EVERYONE can experience the JOY of having a* MOONRISE KINGDOM *kind of BABY.*

End rant.

So when people say something dumb, remind them and yourself that unplanned can be amazing. It can mean that something you never thought about is now open to you. It can shake up your world and fill it with warmth, or at least very cute clothing. It can offer a path you may have never considered, but one in which a more enlightened or healthier truth is at the other end. You may not change everyone's mind, and that's okay, too. You only need to worry about you and your own personal *Moonrise Kingdom.*

8.

IF YOUR FRIENDS AND FAMILY START ACTING LIKE DRAMATIC WEIRDOS

If you are lucky, your surprise pregnancy will find you surrounded by friends and family eager to help, happy to pitch in, over the moon with joy, and more than willing to hang out with you and support you while you do nothing but moan about your expanding ass. But not everyone (ahem, me) decides to be friends with mature, exceptionally thoughtful people ready to drop out of the weekly bar crawl to go crib shopping. What's more, some people will be worse than just indifferent about your breeding; they'll be downright shitty.

And I was all set to talk you through the variety of possible reactions to your surprise pregnancy, not from colleagues and strangers (as we just discussed), but people who actually claim to love you—the shocked parent, the annoyed friend who still wants to party, the offended sister-in-law who has been trying unsuccessfully for years to procreate—but I have decided that it is not worth any more of your time to parse the complex responses of others to your life choices, surprise or not. You're busy. You need peace. You need Zen. You need a field of immunity from bullshit around you. It is not your job to make anyone else but you feel good about this pregnancy.

Anyone who bails on you and your genetically superior baby at this most vulnerable time in your life was just handed the ultimate cosmic loyalty test and failed it harder than a prep at a headbanging contest. But bail they might. The thing about a baby is that you cannot guarantee what it's going to bring out in people, for better or for worse. Babies make people uneasy, frightened, nervous. They remind them of their mortality or the paths they didn't take. For some people, it's a chance to live vicariously through your joy, and, believe you me, that can be just as annoying.

"You never understand life until it grows inside of you."

—Sandra Chami Kassis

Or it's just really awkward. Your normally cool-as-a-cucumber boyfriend might become a nervous wreck now that you're pregnant, taking your temperature every five minutes and asking if you're feeling okay. Or your otherwise caring husband might suddenly become so preoccupied with doomsday prepping that he's completely oblivious to how depressed you've been. Maybe the mother you don't talk to all that much is suddenly trying to show up in your life and be there for you, or the brother you never got along with is mad that you upstaged him and his wife, who wanted to have a baby first. People are sometimes great about babies, but they are also sometimes very weird about babies. Especially if they, too, were totally unprepared for your pregnancy news.

And weirder still is the fact that you are vulnerable enough to need to be cared for, yet you feel yourself getting stronger every day to care for someone else. You are both of these people at once, and sometimes, you will marvel at how often you switch back and forth between being totally helpless and totally together.

The important thing here, no matter how you feel, is that you surround yourself with good people—friends, coworkers, relatives, pets—whose guiding principle during this complicated, exciting, terrifying time in your life is this: You should feel good, not bad, about what you're getting yourself into. Anyone else is persona non grata during this time. Don't fret about this. Make a clean cut where the cutting counts, and embrace what support you have. What may surprise you is that there are tons of people you may not have even been that close to who really enjoy helping you out, for the intrinsic joy of it. Find them, recruit them, lean on them. They are:

Troubleshooters

Troubleshooters are quick on their feet and like to chew on problems and come up with solutions.

Get Their Help With: Organizing and pricing your stuff for a yard sale, putting the crib together, figuring out the best route to the hospital.

Listeners

These are the friends who are good at letting you vent and commiserate.

Get Their Help With: Bitching. When you need to complain, they have a great gripe-worthy angle you haven't even considered yet.

Funny People

Funny people make jokes and see the humor in the unexpected bummers of life.

Get Their Help With: Comic relief in the form of cracking up, laughing at the pain, poking fun at your swelling feet and ever-widening ass, coming up with ridiculous names for your baby.

Planners

Planners are good at doing something you forgot to do, such as think about the future.

Get Their Help With: Figuring out your maternity leave, writing up a birth plan.

Cheerleaders

Best in small doses but very helpful, cheerleaders are always there with a bewilderingly encouraging word or an optimistic take.

Get Their Help With: Birthing classes, especially if you need a partner. These are the people who will remind you that you can totally do this. Because you can do it! They are just somehow naturally good at saying it frequently and convincingly.

Nurturers

These are the intuitive, thoughtful, sympathetic types who just seem to feel for anyone who's struggling.

Get Their Help With: Chatting when you've had an emotional day full of uncertainty or tumultuous feelings.

Cooks

While pregnant, you might be ridiculously, mind-bogglingly hungry. Or, you might vomit at the mere thought of food. If you're the former, anyone who can whip up something tasty that won't give you gestational diabetes is a friend indeed. If you're the latter and you have other mouths to feed at home, this savior can keep them from becoming malnourished.

Get Their Help With: Healthy recipes, low-key dinner parties, office potlucks.

Scavengers

These resourceful folks have a knack for finding things for cheap or free and love the challenge.

Get Their Help With: Tracking down secondhand goods and sweet deals.

While it will never be a happy memory to have distanced yourself from people you thought you'd always be around, it will probably be a big fat relief. Pregnancy is a time of transition. It is a time of release. It is a time of letting go of things to make room for other things, and sometimes those things are people. And when they are very annoying, dramatic, selfish people, they are better released back into the wild. Because there's only room for one dramatic weirdo in this pregnancy: you (or your future child star).

9.

HOW THE HELL DO I GET READY FOR AN ACTUAL BABY?

Great, I'm having a baby! Holy shit, I'm having a baby! If these two sentiments seem contradictory, rest assured they are yin and yang, two parts of the same whole, the good and the bad, the salty and the sweet.

Like planning an office game of Dirty Santa or getting ready for senior prom, you now find yourself suddenly in the precarious position of having to plan for something you weren't exactly ready for. And yet, the logistics and emotional terror of getting your shit together to have an actual baby in your life/house/car/vagina are so abstract as to be almost unimaginable. Sure, you can read about it, conjure it, ask questions about it, but you never have any idea what it will actually be like until it happens directly to your vulva.

So if you find yourself panicking right about now about what lies ahead on the path to preparedness, it's okay. Panic is good! It means your brain is working. Only the undead or heavily medicated are actually cool with massive life changes like this. Your brain, rabid little overthinky beast that it is, is very much alive. It is helping you out, here, in spite of your instinct to remove it wholesale and donate it to a medical curiosities museum.

This is a necessary process. There is an inevitable fear of what we cannot know, an intangible panic in embracing the wild mysterious wonder of human procreation. Broads like us are sure that our uncertainty is showing, so we are extra panicky. We think that we must figure out in nine months' time all the tricks and answers, as if we are searching frantically for that perfect exterior that shows the world we can be mothers after all, even though we did not plan it—*especially* since we did not plan it.

Some questions you might have:

Is this really going to be my life now?
Well it's not going to be someone else's, now, is it?

Who will I be as a mother? How much is this going to change me and all the stuff I was just starting to like about myself?
You'll be the same, but totally different. You'll be the person you've always been, except you just landed on an alien planet for the first time and have to figure it out. Anyone who knows you really well will sense the old you but witness the you-on-the-alien-planet-looking-around-and-processing-it thing. But anyone else will just see a person trying her best.

Am I going to hate being a mother? Because what if I hate it and then I can't take it back?
You can always take it back! Kidding. You can never take this back.

But the good news is that you won't want to. Really. Look, yes, you'll hate parts of it, like the ungodly lack of sleep. Oh, and that thing where you have to be quiet for an entire three hours (while your bladder is slowly imploding) because you're lying quietly next to your baby, who is actually sleeping ever so lightly? And you need this sleep-break, because otherwise you are going to drive everyone off a cliff one by one like a personal cliff chauffeur? That will suck. But unless you're a total jerk—which I suspect you would know before now—you will never, ever actually hate being a mother to your actual child. It will on occasion suck very large balls. But even those balls will taste just like ice cream. If that makes sense.

I already have (x number of) other kid(s)! How can I possibly handle another?

Look at you, O Experienced One! You're ahead of the game. You've already dealt with pregnancy and newborns. What's one more? Okay, it's a big deal, I know. You only have two hands. That's why they invented baby slings and carriers—so you can rein in your mobile children whilst keeping your nonmobile child safe. (And if you have multiple nonmobile children . . . good luck with that.) The truth is, sibling love is overwhelmingly adorable. Plus, it's free labor! Need something from another room? Send your toddler to "help."

I have a full and interesting life. How ever will I make room for this baby?

You'll do it gradually, just like your body gradually makes room for a baby to grow. It squeezes things over and up and around; it expands here, it doubles there, it contracts here. Luckily, you'll have nine months to figure out how your pregnancy will or won't slow you down, and then it's back to square one to see what kind of baby you're having (you're having a baby!?!?!) and how portable or high-maintenance that baby is.

YES! You could have an easy baby or a hard baby, or an in-between baby, or all the kinds of babies in one baby (that's one well-rounded baby). You can't predict it. As if you need a reminder at this point: Don't even bother trying to plan for which kind it is. Babies love nothing more than to poop adorably, but directly, onto your plans.

I'm broke. How can I possibly afford this?

You can't. And when you read some estimates of the overall cost of raising a kid, it's hard to imagine that anyone can, but babies are had and babies are afforded. If you didn't know it before, know this now:

money can be gotten, and often legally. Money may well be the biggest logistical obstacle to push through here, other than the pushing through of the actual baby. You really have to take stock of what you've got (but more likely, don't got) and rethink everything about your current situation, from employment to habitat to spending habits. Don't bother killing yourself sweating a college fund right this second—you'll do that later. Since this pregnancy was a surprise, just think small, bite-size pieces that get you squared away for the baby's birth and those first few months of supplies.

This means make sure you spend the next nine months producing the money to cover living expenses, any hospital bills that won't be covered by insurance, newborn care supplies, and a few weeks off work, if you can swing that. (Do everything you can to swing that—you will never regret it.)

Rethink the following:

Where You Live

If you have to downsize or upsize, do it and do it quickly. The last thing you feel like doing is moving a couch, but wouldn't you rather spend what little free time you have freaking out about the best cloth diaper brand instead of whether you can pay the rent? Or wondering how long a baby can sleep in a dresser drawer?

If you have roommates, great; milk them for all their rent contributions until the baby comes. Just make sure they are the good kind of roommates to be pregnant around, and not the kind who, say, light up a cigarette right next to you after you announce your pregnancy and say, "Shit. What're you gonna do?"

Get this habitat thing squared away as soon as possible. You need a clean, safe place to bring this baby. It does not have to be a big place. Just one free of excessive amounts of cat hair.

Where You Work

If you have a good, stable job and you can swing some maternity leave there, consider sticking with it, even if it's just for the first year of the baby's life, even if it's not your favorite thing ever. You probably don't want to heap more crazy life changes on top of an already crazy one, but that's not to say you shouldn't take a small opportunity you can reap instant rewards from—a quick certification class that means more money, or to jump to a higher-paying position before it's obvious you're prego, which, by the way, is a status you don't have to disclose to any potential employers.

Of course, at some point it will be obvious, so if you plan to change jobs, you might want to do that before the bun is visibly hanging out of the oven. Just consider that the first one in at a new job can be the first one out if layoffs hit, and the only thing worse than being knocked up without any kind of financial plan is being knocked up without a financial plan or a job.

How You Spend Money

Which leads me to this point: Whether or not money is tight, you should now begin to stockpile, stockpile, stockpile, like your life and the life of your unborn child depend on it, because they kind of totally do.

Hold on to any paid time off for after you have the baby, and stop spending unnecessary money. Only spend what you have to! Get more money! How do you do that? Good question.

You:

» **Sell Stuff:** One word: eBay. Two words: Yard sale. More than two words: Can you refinance a car to get a lower monthly payment? Trade in that flashy Mini Cooper for a trusty old used Honda? This is a great time to take stock of all those quirky vintage valuables you've been hoarding and trade them in for diapers, formula, a hospital-grade breast pump, a comfortable maternity wardrobe, a crib, etc. Keep what's irreplaceable, but save the majority of your can't-buy-me-love sentiment for the baby.

» **Quit Going Out:** Cutting out smoking, drinking, and all the attendant costs of dining out saved my husband and me an insane, embarrassing, and incredibly helpful $700 a month. Luckily, I didn't feel much like doing any of those things once I was with child, and the sheer exhaustion of pregnancy alone may make you feel like staying in and watching reruns of *Ally McBeal*. Cook at home, get slothy, and nest.

» **Consider Cloth Diapers:** You don't need much to take care of a newborn, but you do need diapers. Well, there is a diaper-free movement, but that requires that you live in San Francisco and earn more than a quarter of a million dollars annually. The rest of us wannabe progressives will have to settle for old-fashioned cloth diapers. The good news is, they are much improved from the giant safety pin–fastened table napkin of yore.

For an initial investment of a few hundred dollars for starter packs, you can swing cloth diapers for the first year or two of the baby's life (although huge babies tend to out-poop them pretty quickly). You can always supplement with disposables for when you're on the go, but if you want to cut back on costs for diapering by a good third, this is the way to go, whether you're a hippie or not. (Just kidding. Remember, "true" hippies go diaper-free.) Please note that this is only easier (and ultimately, kinder) if you live somewhere with your own washer and dryer. Hauling literally shitty diapers to a communal washer and dryer is a unique form of torture for you and me and everyone around us.

» **Consider Nursing:** It ain't always fun, convenient, or easy, but it is free. Well, mostly free. The associated costs with nursing are not much compared to formula feeding. That would include the nursing bras, which can be gotten secondhand or on the cheap, and the pumping equipment if you are back at work and someone else will be feeding the baby breast milk via bottle. Pumping equipment includes a pump, bottles, a storage system like plastic bags, and, of course, a refrigerator/freezer—so, not such a great idea if you're a freegan vagrant. Keep in mind you'll be hungrier, or what I call

Pregzilla, while nursing, as it requires a few more calories than even pregnancy. Which means a slightly higher grocery bill. Still way cheaper than formula.

» **Exploit the Baby Shower:** I was pretty *meh* about the baby shower, as I'm not a fan of forced small talk and dumb games, until I realized that I could get almost all the gear I needed for the baby's first year in terms of gadgets and clothes. (Keep in mind that you usually only need about half of what those online suggestion lists would have you believe!) So I sat through two hours of yawn with people I liked, but also with people who I only sorta liked.

Exploit away, and keep those receipts. It's hard to say what you'll need most for your baby until you get into your own routine, but again, it's less than you think. You need, at bare minimum, only five or six basic outfits, plus stuff to sleep in. Socks. Hats. Layers, depending on the season. You do not need baby shoes until your child is walking. You will probably use every onesie and baby blanket you ever get, and a basic grooming kit with a nasal bulb, thermometer, soft brush, and infant nail trimmers will be super useful. But if that vibrating chair doesn't work for your baby, trade it for the jumpy swing your kid will love. A crib is useful at first, even if you end up doing the Family Bed—every baby needs a baby jail to go to. So buy one (new and cheap or secondhand and cheaper) after you research the cheapest, safest up-to-date one on the market.

» **Use Secondhand Stuff:** Once word is out that you're pregnant, you'll have a gaggle of parents with older kids looking to unload on you every old car seat (make sure you can trust/verify that it has never been in an accident or been recalled, and is not more than three years old), bouncy seat, baby bathtub, newborn book, and rattle they haven't had the time or courage to let go of. Take it! Take it all. You'll buy your own special keepsake items for your baby, too, but in the meantime, you will save big by reusing other people's stuff at no cost to you, and becoming part of the great giant oneness of parenting hand-me-downs. Pass them on when you're done, and you keep the circle going. This is so great for toys, because newborns literally can't tell if they are playing with a wooden spoon or a $300 Tiffany's rattle.

With these tips, there's no reason you can't square away the logistics of money and stuff you need to have a baby and focus on freaking out about the rest of it. When in doubt, just remember these suspiciously simple yet totally true words of wisdom, passed down from mother to mother to mother: *Somehow, it just all works out.*

I remember when a mother I worked with told me that. I thought she sounded like some kind of cliché Stepford wife, passing along some trite little tidbit to ease my worry. But it was true. Somehow, with no money and no stability, we turned it all around and set ourselves up for the least amount of financial worry possible that first year. And sometimes, you discover that the thing you were most worried about not being able to cover is not a problem after all.

In our case, that was the hospital bill. We had calculated that with my insurance coverage, our personal liability in hospital costs might still be as much as $3,000 all said and done. What we didn't realize was that a federal law requires an insurance company to cover a newborn under both parents' policies. So even though my husband had just gotten a new job with insurance that had not even kicked in, we were suddenly double covered, and our total bill to have a baby at a reputable, upstanding university hospital, including all the gyno visits, was a whopping $300.

And as crazy-making as it all might feel, somehow, while you are chasing down all these loose ends, you find a kind of peaceful balance taking over. A kind of calm. A kind of serene self-containment. As you are intellectually freaking about logistics, something—hormones?—seems to say, this is all just as it should be. Just be in the state you are in. It is the beginning of not so much freaking out but instead marveling at what your brain and your body are capable of doing for you and for your baby.

And then, slowly but surely, you realize you are getting used to this being pregnant thing. You reach for the brass ring. You will pep-talk the shit out of this when you need to. You will learn to say a series of things to yourself, when you get overwhelmed with exhaustion and feelings and the money hasn't all come together just yet, that will make you feel like you're in a pretty cool war movie and have a pain-in-the-ass sergeant barking motivations at you: *Remember your training, soldier! This is bigger than you! You can do this!*

You really can. Nope, this isn't what you or I thought would happen, if we were thinking at all, but this is what has happened, and we've chosen it. We waddle straight into our new reality, even if we have to sometimes grab onto a very wobbly handrail.

10.

HOW TO EAT ALL THE STUFF YOU AREN'T SUPPOSED TO

Is there really a whole bunch of stuff you can't eat while pregnant? Or is it just some Orwellian mind control? Doesn't it feel even more punishing when you had no real intention of doing this in the first place? Either way, pregnancy is an almost Zen-like challenge for a woman where what she does is suddenly equally as important as what she does not do. Where what she wants is in direct opposition to what she needs, but with enough guilt to cover all possible feelings in between.

None of this is as painfully obvious as when it comes to your dietary and consumption requirements. Upside: It's not like anyone gives you some crazy, fascist list and tells you exactly what you can and can't do. Downside: For the love of God, why won't anyone just give you a crazy, fascist list so you know what you can and can't do?! (Warning: While you are out in the world navigating this imaginary list of what you can and cannot do/consume, it feels like everyone else in the world has that exact same list in their back pocket and is at the ready to pull it out and slap you upside the belly with it at a moment's notice.)

The thing about pregnancy and dietary restrictions, though, is that the list of stuff you allegedly can't eat isn't really all that long. It's just that when you suddenly have a list of stuff you allegedly can't eat, it seems like it contains all the most delicious, tantalizing food in the world—bonus bitching rights if you are a sushi-loving, unpasteurized cheese–eating alcoholic, and who isn't? Here are the biggest surprises I encountered as I navigated eating right for nine months, and tips for getting around them.

Alcohol

Understatement of the year: My relationship to drinking changed when I got pregnant. And then it changed again. At first, I would have vomited at the mere thought of the stuff, but then again, I'd have vomited at the thought of anything. By the time I hit my second and third trimesters, I swung 180 degrees the other way, and it was tough to face another Friday night at home without much to take the edge off. My doctor sort of made it easier when he told me he could not guarantee that any amount of alcohol consumption during pregnancy was safe, so he would not condone its use. I was all resigned to that when my pregnant boss said her doctor told her that it was totally fine if she had a glass of wine at night during her pregnancy. WTF, y'all? Surely the truth is somewhere in the middle.

The Workaround: Find another doctor, or move to Europe. Okay, so more realistic options include combining those two competing pieces of medical wisdom from my doctor and my boss in my head and deciding that if once every couple of weeks I had a glass of wine, I could live with myself.

Also: I just thought about France, where pregnant women are told to limit the booze to no more than two drinks during pregnancy. A day. Over the course of my pregnancy, I had maybe five or six glasses of wine total to strike a boozy balance. I do recommend doing this at home, alone, under the sheets with a flashlight, though, instead of, say, choosing to partake in a glass of wine at the office Christmas party, where you will be straight-up scowled at by a table of do-gooders as if you are auditioning for a show called *Riskiest Pregnancy Ever, Stupid Edition.*

Deli Meat

I knew I'd be finger-wagged away from alcohol, but I was genuinely surprised that I'd have to go cold turkey on cold turkey—literally. You're not supposed to eat deli meat while pregnant because of the risk of the bacteria listeria. If you're not a fan of deli sandwiches, this may hardly seem like a sacrifice, but for those of us who love nothing more than a few thin slices of turkey for a snack or on a salad, it's a terrible drag.

The Workaround: All you have to do is buy the stuff that's nitrate- and nitrite-free and nuke it till it steams to kill any potential bacteria. It's not cold anymore, duh, but it'll do. By the end of my pregnancy I wanted nothing more than cold deli meat for weeks on end, but for those months when it was hot turkey or no turkey, you could find me standing directly around the corner from the microwave while my husband steamed a plate for me.

Sushi

Ask your doctor about sushi, the pregnancy "don't" that will leave you terrified of even the friendliest Hawaiian roll. No, really, ask your doctor whether it's ACTUALLY a no-go on sushi consumption during pregnancy, or if you should just avoid raw mollusks and shellfish. Discuss the fact that sushi is only sometimes raw fish, but it has typically been flash frozen, which kills any parasites. And hello? Japanese women aren't exactly avoiding this mainstay of their diet during gestation.

But if your doctor still convinces you that it's actually a greater worry than you'd realized and backs it up with some science, unless you feel like getting a really fast medical degree to debate her, eat it at your own risk. Also: new claims that most of the fish used in sushi are mislabeled, and could actually be full of mercury, is not doing sushi any favors.

The Workaround: Eat sushi if you like, just get the many types of cooked fish found in California rolls or Rainbow rolls. Ask your server. Or, if you feel confident about raw fish, be mindful of the prep conditions and only patronize restaurants with perfect health scores—

this should be a goal all the time, but especially while pregnant, because who wants morning sickness AND food poisoning? Also, definitely avoid high-mercury fish that you weren't going to eat anyway, like shark and tilefish, which approximately zero people I know have ever eaten (on purpose). You can also eat tuna, or imitation, fully cooked crabmeat.

Cheese

You're not supposed to eat soft cheese when pregnant due to the same risk of listeria that deli meat poses. That means goodbye Brie, goodbye unpasteurized French cheeses made from raw milk.

The Workaround: Just like the cold turkey solution, you can eat Brie if it's heated, which happens to be a very popular dish. Raw milk cheeses aged for longer than sixty days are supposed to be A-OK—check with your doctor. And what's to stop you from loading up on good, old-fashioned pasteurized Cheddar, mozzarella, pepperjack, and a host of other totally pedestrian cheeses that pose no risk? Only constipation and looking like a philistine.

Spicy Food

The no-no for hitting the hot zone of spices seems to be based on old wives' tales of "spotty skin" in babies whose mothers ate spicy foods—or that wicked heartburn.

The Workaround: If you're craving spicy foods, eat spicy foods. This will feel super great once you're staring down the third trimester with your stomach now located directly behind your tongue. If the heartburn starts showing up, go for the mildest version of spicy food you can, er, stomach, which is zero. And embrace TUMS. Or, some people recommend faking yourself out by just having something a little salty every now and then.

Raw Cookie Dough

I was never one of those fanatical raw cookie dough people, thank God, but guess what I wanted to eat more than ever once I knew I couldn't have it? Raw cookie dough. Obviously, raw eggs are the culprit here, and for good reason: who wants to name their baby Salmonella?

The Workaround: Duh, *cooked* cookie dough, a.k.a. cookies. Crumble them up and sprinkle them over ice cream for a terrible, ghastly alternative to eating it raw. Just don't overdo it, because gestational diabetes puts you at real risk for premature babies and other complications. Man, *nothing* about pregnancy is stress-free.

Aversions

For all the stuff you supposedly can't eat, the real excitement begins when you discover all the stuff you don't want to eat because it suddenly seems so disgusting it makes you want to die. Case in point for me: chicken. What was once the most benign, boring food on the block suddenly became so revolting to me that I couldn't even smell it without wanting to hurl. This lasted my entire pregnancy and was annoying because I was trying to save money, and chicken is about the cheapest meat out there for those of us unwilling to kill our own opossum.

The Workaround: Try to avoid the offending food (which will suddenly appear everywhere you look, including your dreams). I suppose I could have eaten fake vegetarian chicken, but even this was too chicken-like for me. I just had to not eat it, and luckily I didn't actually want to. Instead, we went with lean red meats or lean pork chops or lamb, and focused on really filling vegetarian dishes with lentils and black beans. Eventually, I got my chicken groove back, about six months after the baby was born, when I was thrilled to be back to being bored by chicken.

. . .

Once you've subbed out all the naughty foods for perfectly nice ones, you will definitely be bored, you will totally still crave offending foods to an almost unreal degree, but as so many pregnancy-related victories go, you can at least finally enjoy something even better than cold turkey sushi dessert surprise: becoming even more smug, self-satisfied, and self-congratulatory about the sacrifices you've made for your child than ever before. You have no idea how handy this will come in later as a future attendee of the playgrounds and preschools of the world.

11.

EVERYTHING IS BEAUTIFUL
(in Its Own Disgusting Way):
A PUBLIC SERVICE RANT

As a woman, I've been told some pretty top-shelf lies in my lifetime—that I should totally try a dark spray tan, that gaucho pants are a good idea for my body type, that a guy at a bar offering air conditioning and steaks back at his place is THE guy to go home with—but nothing holds a candle to the grand myth that pregnancy is some beautiful, wondrous thing.

Sure, the concept is beautiful—miracle of life, human oneness, yadda yadda yadda. Even the most unexpected pregnancy will make you marvel at the power of creation at some point or another. But the physical part, what actually happens to your hair, face, body, and hormones? Notsomuch.

FYI: Pregnancy is nature, and nature is gross. Nature is wet things, oozing things, morphing things, decaying things. It is things pushing things out while sucking other things in. It is fermenting and bubbling things, stretchy and gooey things. It is things hitching onto other things for a ride. It is all these things wrapped up into a big, bright, dark, fresh, disgusting, clean, wondrous mess. It's science, and science is not cute.

Per the usual for women, however, when you are experiencing this scientific mess via your own body, you are supposed to still be all cute about it. Ludicrous. Well, here is my public service announcement. You do NOT have to be all cute about it. Even if you feel, as I did, like Gumby with a beer gut. ESPECIALLY if you feel like Gumby with a beer gut. Make no mistake, though: It's not cause for a shame spiral—it's natural, after all. It is cause, rather, for a triumphant wallow.

To wit: You are under no obligation to suddenly make more of an effort to flat-iron your hair, embrace florals, or take lots of showers. You need not emanate rainbows and sunshine. You need not glow with vanilla-scented warmth or emanate brown sugar–scrub radiance. You need not make other women feel better about themselves, their bodies, having babies, or not having babies through your own pregnancy. You need not remind grandmothers of their brood, mothers of their past pregnancies, or fathers of their fates. Just be you. Just be pregnant. Whatever that feels like. For you. On whatever day it is. Hey, if that's a darling, glowing, chipper whiff of fresh-cut flowers, good on ya.

For me, it was like suddenly inhabiting the body of a seal. A very smelly, greasy, tired, uncomfortable, and really super pregnant seal. Maybe twice a month I would feel good, somehow finding a maternity shirt that didn't look like I was a seal who had done acid in a Casual Corner design workshop. Those days, it was very comforting and marvelous to be pregnant. Most other days, I was far too slumberingly sluggish to be bothered, and it showed.

Yup, I got fat—the quitting drinking and smoking made me gain weight faster than compound interest on a payday loan, above and beyond the recommended 25 to 30 pounds. I'm not calling my specifically baby-related weight gain *fat*. That part was all normal and tolerable—the bump swells like a little pouch, and your boobs become gigantic cantaloupes. It was the extra stuff that killed me: the rapid padding of the thighs and arms that made me want to roll around in a swimming pool and bounce a beach ball off my nose.

> **"I just started calling myself Swamp Ass. Like, I have 'swamp ass' right now. I had major swamp ass because I was wearing these Spanx to hold in my gut. It's like the bayou up in that region."**
>
> —Jessica Simpson

Then, things got a little, how shall I say . . . zitty? Sweaty. Smelly. I smelled like pee from all the literal peeing on myself thanks to the pressure on my bladder. About halfway through my pregnancy, I pretty much stopped taking showers because I was so uncomfortable standing for very long. That's right! I was a big, fat, zitty, greasy, pee-smelly, unwashed lumbering seal.

The weird thing? As much as I hated it, I also loved it.

Here's why: How often do women get a free pass on how they look? The answer is never, not even when senile. I like to helpfully point out that if there's ever a time to smash and grab your way out of the oppressive heat of grooming and really learn how to let go, pregnancy is it. (Also, the first two years of the baby's life, but that's another matter.)

That doesn't mean that anyone else is likely to support this celebration of the muckier side of the muck, however. Each day, as this sea otter rolled into work, I could hear what people were asking huffily in their heads, and with great irritation, as they gave me the once-over.

"You know you can still be cute while pregnant, right?" they harrumphed.

But really they were thinking, *Oh God, how bad could it be if you don't even want to still look cute?!?!?*

I'd say medium-bad. Just short of psychotic. Sorry, kids, but bloating and heartburn and a surprise revisited childhood (emotionally) are hard to make look cute on a Friday night, no matter what handbag you're carrying. Add to that the hormonal surges that could take out a city block and, well, they don't call pregnant ladies Oozing Hormonal Shapeshifters for nothing. (Technically, no one calls them that but me.)

All this bio-horror might be fine if you'd had any warning; all of it could be just great if there weren't any of the pressure to put a fat 'n' happy spin on it, or to actually smile your way through that much polyester-blended floral. But no, there everyone is, rooting for you to waddle optimistically around with a glowy complexion and a perfectly symmetrical baby bump so . . . what? They can feel good about themselves?

And therein lies the (belly) rub: Not only did no one tell you the potential for such grossness during gestation—that for nine months you might feel like a swelling, ailing [insert large water animal of your choice] participating in a medical study about ailing [insert large water animal of your choice] who smells so bad that no one wants to be friends with them—no one told you that you will also inadvertently become An Informal Representative of Pregnancy to the General Public.

Like the pregnancy equivalent of running for local political office or heading up a book club, everyone's now looking at you to see how you'll be portraying capital-B Breeding. Will you make it look hard? Easy? Dreadful? Disgusting? Elegant?

For the unplanned pregnancy, this is quadruple the tap-dance difficulty level. Not only did you have no desire to hand over the keys to your body to the physical equivalent of a reckless teenager, but you're also likely to be struggling enough as it is to set your emotional fears aside. Here you are, dealing with all these intense emotional and physical, um, issues, and these barbaric jerkwads want you to make sure you've brushed your hair.

What's more, the grossness is somehow proportional: The more disgusting it is for you to be pregnant, the worse everyone else seems to vibe you for it. That's right: Your suffering somehow signals others that you're violating your end of the pregnant social contract, which apparently includes making sure being pregnant looks 100-percent joyful.

While we all certainly wish we could embody the glowy perfection of life pulsing within, some of us come a lot closer to nasty *South Park* bus driver Veronica Crabtree instead.

Now that I've exonerated you from having to portray perfection, let me tell you this: It's really not *all* bad. The fullness, the kicking-ness, the aliveness, the gestating-ness. There is a kind of serene self-containment that comes along with it, and at times it can feel like full femininity in bloom, and extremely beautiful.

And even for every way that it can be terrible, it is also pretty terrific. For me, there were a couple of very specific upsides to the experience, aside from more opened doors and the chance to do less work at work. In one way, I got physically closer to my husband, believe it or not.

One morning, a few months into the pregnancy, I woke up with extreme pain in both ears. They both felt hot and throbbing deep inside, and I wondered what weird infection had befallen me that would cause such binaural distress.

My husband, an audio engineer who is obsessed with sound to the extent that he will routinely go off on tangents about everything from how often microphones are incorrectly positioned on TVs (answer: constantly) to proper ear care, said he would take a look at them. He is the sort of guy who also happens to have a headlamp lying around. Or four.

He clicked the bright light on and peered into my ear canal while I sat there, cringing.

"Gross," he said. Then a pause.

"Gross what?" I asked fearfully.

"You have a monster zit," he said, then moved to the other side to take a look. "In both ears."

I pictured volcanoes of throbbing heat in my head. Both zits were in way too far for me to do anything about them myself, but the pressure was killing me. So, for the next week, each night he took turns sterilizing a needle, puncturing the swollen mounds and pressing gently down on them with an alcohol-dipped cotton swab, which always elicited a soft, padded popping sound, followed by warm oozing. Then he followed up with a cooling dab of hydrogen peroxide. (I would not recommend doing this on your own at home unless you just happen to be married to a Boy Scout.)

Somehow, it was tremendously satisfying for the both of us to perform this relieving ritual, and we joked about how it had been, without a doubt, more intimate than any sex either of us had ever had.

Which leads me to the other upside. In the middle of the trash heap grossathon, around the middle of the second trimester, the hormones shifted into inexplicable overdrive, and suddenly I was hornier than I had ever been in my life. My husband could have run screaming off a cliff, but he emphatically did not. Cue the beautiful.

We had sex in the morning, sex in the afternoon on lunch breaks, and sex at night. We had sex in the shower and sex on the couch. The sex was exactly how you would imagine sex if you felt completely uninhibited and completely free from any fear of silliness, judgment, or impropriety. It was all about desire, and zero about how I looked.

Positions changed fluidly; desire swelled along with appropriate sexual organs. Aside from having to stop occasionally for overheating, it was good, old-fashioned marathon sex.

But that's not all! It was death row sex, it was bon voyage sex, it was European-vacation-with-the-hot-Italian-guy-you'll-never-see-again sex. It was *Before Sunrise* and *Before Sunset* with all the bulging anticipation in between.

If there is a beauty in pregnancy, perhaps it is an ironic one. Somehow, in spite of all the worst, most uncomfortable physical changes I'd endured, including adolescence, I had never felt so free and light in my life as I did when we were having this crazy-good sex. It made all the ugliness and discomfort melt away like so many pats of butter. Mmmm. Butter.

It also allowed me to have fun with all the awkwardness. Perhaps all the sex was making me giddy, but each day, as I shuffled back into the newspaper office where I worked as a new and improved sea otter with a glow of my own, and plopped into my cubicle next to the two twenty-something dudes I'd recruited for the music section, it was a never-ending slapstick with me as the star, and I found a way to laugh off all the ill-fitting suffocation of my pregnant, alien-feeling body.

For some reason, I found it immensely satisfying to hike one leg up onto a chair, rub my belly, and make a grunting/seething kind of Igor-inspired noise. "Heeeeeeee," I would seethe and rub with one leg hiked up.

"Dude, for some reason that makes me feel really weird," said a twenty-something writer named Patrick who sat at the next cube, shaking his head and backing away.

"I know," I would respond with glee. "That's the point."

And that's my point to you, friend. Raising a child may take a village. But while you're pregnant, you can make that village suffer along with you. Hey, it's the least you can do for all the lies they told you.

12.

WHAT NOT TO WEAR, UNPLANNED PREGNANCY EDITION

What you need to wear to weather this Kafkaesque transformation depends entirely on how well you're physically weathering it.

Are you already one of those cute people with a cute sense of fashion, and/or a rich person with access to well-made, durable but chic maternity wear made of luxurious fabrics? Who happens to have a totally symmetrical baby bump? If so, you don't need my help.

Are you, on the other hand, one of those people who barely has it together as it is, and probably won't be able to keep it together physically either, and whose emotional state leaves you in perpetual hoodie mode? Do you often forget showers or find daily showerers to be suspiciously groomed? Do you kinda hate consumerism and loathe shopping? Would you look cute, maybe, if someone would do all the shopping and work for you, but barring that, you're shit out of luck? Does your baby bump look like it's a half watermelon with a banana bunch on the side?

Then you've come to the right place. Let's get you sorted out.

You may be staring down an unplanned pregnancy, but we can't have you doing that looking like some kind of crazy bag lady muttering about maternity leave policies. Just as you've worked to wrangle your emotions into something resembling basic sanity, so must you present to the world a picture of presentable somewhat togetherness. Save your breakdowns for the shower, or better yet, gyno visits and birthing classes, where there are the highest concentrations of qualified and financially compensated professionals to help you through them.

What you'll need are a few key maternity items with enough variety to keep your office's emotional vulnerability hounds from sniffing 'round your cubicle all the time trying to determine your breaking point. You'll need to look competent and maybe even somewhat professional at times. Mostly, you'll want to look like you aren't batshit crazy simply because you're unexpectedly pregnant and still haven't figured out how to swing the hospital bill.

(A note about finances: I'm not assuming you're broke, just that perhaps you aren't sitting on a maternity wear pregnancy fund and don't have a ton of dough earmarked for this occasion.)

What really stuck in my craw about dressing for pregnancy was that the need for actual maternity wear occurred so early in the pregnancy. I thought I had at least a couple of months of wearing my same old duds until I'd have to break down and buy polyester, when instead, in a matter of weeks I could no longer button my jeans. (A friend told me the Bella Band was terrific, but that friend was a liar, and the Bella Band was about as effective in helping me keep on my regular jeans as a garter belt on Godzilla.) I had to act fast, yet while moving very sluggishly, to procure a wardrobe that fit.

The problem was, so much of what I encountered was so the fundamental opposite of my current style, much less of everything I looked for in comfortable clothing: florals, big patterns, bold colors, wacky designs—like something your average Southern Baptist organist would wear to a Wednesday night church hoedown. Sure, you can find plain T-shirts and khakis, but if you're looking for anything beyond that, things get dicey, fast. The patterns that would look delightful in a normal size are suddenly outrageous when printed on the amount of fabric needed for a maternity shirt.

I was a, ahem, journalist, okay? And a fan of rock 'n' roll? Take Me Seriously, Please, I broadcast to the world. I Am a Woman, but I'm Still a Person, Too, and a Cool One at That, I pleaded to the indifferent racks. No, Really, I'm Too Smart to Be Consumed with Trivial Matters Such as Fashion, I tried again. Which meant I owned two good pairs of skinny black jeans, a lot of flats, and a variety of shirts in solid earth tones.

So it was almost more alarming than the pregnancy itself when I also discovered that maternity wear is ultra-feminine, ultra-flirty, ultra-fun, or ultra-frumpy and downright matronly. And I couldn't have felt less feminine during my first trimester already, in no small part because I was transmogrifying into a walrus faster than I could say "merengue." Lacy stuff, eyelets, beads, and baubles abounded. Was I pregnant or going salsa dancing? While wearing a doily?

A fiscal word of warning: Maternity stuff isn't all that much cheaper than regular clothes, in spite of the fact that it's obviously temporary and somewhat disposable by design, given that most of us are only pregnant for nine months. Sometimes it's actually *more* expensive. Sure, it uses more fabric and is specialty wear, which may justify the markup in the manufacturer's mind, but this tactic would never fly with plus sizes at typical retail stores.

Sadly, the exploitation of the world's poorer economies and workers will have to be quietly pushed to the bottom of your list of things you really were going to stop patronizing yet again this year while you try to navigate your own personal American travesty.

That burden dubiously lifted, there are a number of totally affordable places making somewhat decent maternity wear that almost any budget can accommodate. There really are things for $10 or less, and most of them last at least a few weeks, so long as it isn't all that windy out.

No joke: Brands such as Old Navy, H&M, and Gap make (mostly) serviceable maternity wear. Sure, sometimes you'll wonder if it was put together with duct tape and Popsicle sticks. I recommend that you find a few well-made pieces to last the long haul, namely jeans and a good dress. It will feel good and be worth the money if you can swing it. I wore a black pair of skinny maternity jeans (sartorial dissonance?) from the beginning right up to the bitter end, and nervously dropped $110 to do it. I still got 'em, though; the seams are shredded and the fabric has become translucent, but I'll never forget what they did for me and my oddly shaped baby bump.

Depending on your job, the season, and your current lifestyle, you'll need to invest in a few basics. Here are some key items:

» Two decent pairs of jeans.
» A couple of comfy, stretchy yoga-type maternity pants.
» Tank tops galore.
» A variety of T-shirts in a variety of colors.
» A few printed tops for "color."
» One kickin' maxi dress.
» One stretchy cotton skirt.
» Leggings, leggings, leggings.
» Shorts: Are you insane?
» At least two good bras and at least a week's worth of comfy cotton underwear: Be prepared to spend your entire budget here. Seriously. Heave-ho.
» A maternity bathing suit: For the bold and the beautiful, or anyone who just doesn't give a fuck.

If you feel like your bottom half is . . . oddly shaped, choose dark colors that minimize that part of your body. You could also wear scoop-neck tops in prints you can stand to accentuate your boobs, which by now will be the headline of every story you're telling whether you like it or not.

In spite of what I've implied here, maternity clothes *can* look lovely, and I would never suggest that the pregnant body isn't beautiful. I think it is, at least on other people. I saw so many women who looked really gorgeous while pregnant. And of course I've definitely seen it happen in pictures. Magazines mostly. And sure, I've seen loads of actual women in person look extremely cute in maternity wear, women who seem to have proportional pregnant bellies that make some kind of structural, biological sense. (Nevermind how good the women who model maternity wear look. Did you notice they aren't actually pregnant?)

If you're comfortable and able, forget all this advice and just do what I never had the guts to do: Wear PJs every single day. If you can pull this off, you are my hero. Plz send pics. But for those who are not interested in turning your pregnancy into a conceptual art project, go forth armed with a casual array of comfortable clothes that will let you look like the best gently expanding you that you can be.

13.

YOUR NEW BOYFRIEND: FOOD

One minute you are staring at a positive pregnancy test, and nine months later you've gained 80 pounds, gotten a terrible haircut, and now look like a pregnant pageboy. No, it's not a nightmare; it's a super-true pregnancy story plucked from one of my friends, who at the bitter end of her gestation gained so much weight that she had to rock back and forth to get off the toilet.

I wasn't far behind her. By the end of my pregnancy I weighed 209 pounds, 60 pounds heavier than where I'd started. Looking back, I can scarcely remember where the weight had come from, only that it had felt like it piled on mercilessly, the universe willing the pounds to occupy my body against all protest.

How do we end up here? No one starts a pregnancy, no matter how unexpected, planning on ballooning to comical, toilet-rocking proportions, to say nothing of that unfortunate mistake of getting a drastic haircut in your final trimester. And yet many women gain far more than the 25 to 35 pounds that are considered a safe weight gain. The answer is obvious: HELLO, unplanned pregnancy + can't go out + hormonal upheaval = emotional eating. In other words, your new boyfriend is food.

This happens to women who plan their pregnancies as well, no doubt, as food is probably the greatest pregnancy temptation outside of marrying anyone capable of a halfway decent back rub. But those of us who are ambushed by pregnancy feel even less prepared for how hard it will be to stop self-soothing the burn with a very romantic bag of chips. Is that really such a bad thing? Think of the advantages of a food affair:

» **It offers endless variety.** Your real boyfriend/husband/partner is working every day for a lot of hours, and with the same haircut he has always had. Food is different. It's mysterious. It's transformative. One minute, it's cottage cheese and blueberries and the next minute it's magically a slice of cheeseless with whole-wheat crust. See? You just got hungry for a variety boyfriend made of whole-wheat crust.

» **It doesn't talk back.** Your husband is wondering if you're going to get up and go for a nice walk today instead of watching yet another nonstop season of *Teen Mom,* which always makes you blubber ridiculously for hours. But this bowl of steel-cut oatmeal with pecans and a tiny smidge of agave likes *Teen Mom.* A lot. Let's plow through, it says, because I can't wait to see what happens to Amber in season three.

» **It likes you just as you are.** Have you ever heard a plate of lightly sea-salted cucumber slices complain about the way you clean a bathroom? Noooooooooo. It doesn't care about hygiene. Fruit salad cannot smell your pits, and if it could, it would LOVE them. Truth. Food is the Mark Darcy to your Bridget Jones. Swoon.

» **It doesn't mind hearing your stories over and over again.** The only thing steamed broccoli loves more than being baked in a red pepper gratin is hearing for the hundredth time about the first time you discovered Jane Austen.

» **It wants to be with you forever-ever.** Greek yogurt and raspberries with wheat germ loves you for you. And he'd like to stick around for as long as you'll have him.

Of course, there's a hot, tasty problem with thinking this way. It's called weight gain. And contrary to what all depictions of pregnancy everywhere ever have claimed, "eating for two" while preggers does not mean eating for two complete humans. It's you, and this second living thing the size of a goldfish or a tiny lizard. Do you know what lizards eat? One bug a week. In human terms, that's about 300 calories worth of extra bugs every day, or approximately three-fourths of a Starbucks blueberry muffin.

Hopefully, you're reading this a) before you finished the muffin, b) before you gained the maximum 35 pounds considered safe weight gain for a pregnancy, and c) after your morning sickness eases up, because I did just write about eating bugs and all.

So what now? Obviously you want to strike a balance somewhere between eating healthy and getting through nine months of discomfort. Now let's put our heads together and figure this one out and keep your food boyfriend.

» **Eat well most of the time.** Sad tromboooooone. This seems like it would go without saying, but I wish someone had said that to me every day of my pregnant life. There are great nutrition plans online that can help you figure out a more realistic way to feel full without going overboard, and you should use them (says the person who gained 60 pounds and never found those diet plans because she was too busy feeling emotional). Of course, gestational diabetes or a nutrient-deprived fetus is no one's idea of a cool Facebook status update, so like a decent soon-to-be mother, try to eat more nutritious and well-rounded meals. This will also be good practice for eventually feeding a child, whom you will want to eat more than just cake pops on the daily.

» **If you're going to go overboard, eat too much of a good thing, at least.** Sure, this logic can probably be easily undone—more of anything is still more calories—but I still submit that if you're absolutely going crazy and feel you must keep eating, keep eating fresh fruit, or cottage cheese, or a handful of nuts. They are less likely to have the insane calories of another piece of pie or a second muffin, and you get to feel approximately 25 percent less guilt.

» **Do other stuff.** Distraction works. If you're still hungry and you've blown past your daily allowance of calories, you're going to have to get busy nesting or just relax away from food.

» **Exercise.** It felt really good to walk during pregnancy, and when I wasn't walking, there was an entire trimester when I was extremely horny and wanted sex constantly.

» **Don't revert to bad habits**. I super really truly wanted to smoke the whole time I was pregnant, but I wasn't going to. It wasn't even an option. There was just absolutely no way I was going to smoke during my pregnancy. Not even once, no matter how glamorous the magazines make it look. Okay, so I'm only talking about that one controversial photo shoot in French *Vogue*, but STILL.

» **Go easy on yourself.** If you find yourself hitting the cottage cheese and peaches more times than makes sense, don't beat yourself up about it. If the choice is to smoke or eat some more cottage cheese and peaches, let's just say everyone is happy I picked the peaches. Perhaps my thighs to this day are not happy about it, but we've worked out a deal where they aren't allowed to see any sunlight.

» **Don't buy the really bad stuff.** Just make it easier on yourself and shop the perimeter of the supermarket, and make snacks that are healthy. And bank on the fact that at a certain point, you won't feel like getting off the couch anyway, thereby eventually ending the grocery store reign of terror.

» **Enlist a friend to help.** Do not make friends with the enabler who will shoot cupcakes into your mouth out of a T-shirt cannon. Find the good friend who will bring you the plate of cucumber slices and razz you about why you wanted the cupcakes again anyway.

» **Get used to eating like you're in the Witness Protection Program.** People are into watching people eat, especially pregnant women. It's really annoying how much interest people may show in what's going into your mouth, especially under the guise of "concern" for your health. Instead, do your indulgent eating like you drink your wine: under the covers with a flashlight, like everyone else. Give them nothing!

» **Realize it's a very short affair.** The good news is that he is totally available to you 24/7 during this most emotionally vulnerable time. The bad news is that he is a bad boyfriend, unreliable, up to no good, and always manipulating you into doing things you shouldn't.

Yes, a serious relationship with food is nothing to sneeze at, but not because it should be your boyfriend. Because that would ruin the food. Break up with him now, before he becomes your husband. You can't raise a baby with a casserole.

14.

HOW TO DEAL WITH EMOTIONAL UPHEAVAL

Your mom was kind of a hosebeast. Your sister was always copying you. Your dad didn't "get" you, and your friends were pretty much wildebeests disguised as hyenas disguised as jackals. Disguised as jackanapes. (Apparently, there's lotsa scavenging and foraging going on in your life.) Real or not, it suddenly feels like everything bad that ever happened to you comes back up faster than a case of pregnant heartburn. And guess what? It all sucks.

Is it pre-partum depression? Fetus blues? Procreating crazies? Why is it happening to you? Does it even matter? Because whether it is a completely hormonally invented nadir or merely proof that you failed to properly resolve your most deep-seated issues, it is time for you to act out your own version of an afterschool special, replete with a banged-up station wagon and some mousy brown hair. And when you weren't planning on being pregnant (and maybe because of it), when this emotional baggage hits, it hits hard, like posting a Facebook selfie that garners exactly zero Likes.

Part of you is happy. Part of you is sad. Most of you is happily sad and sadly happy all at once for nearly this whole nine months (and, sorry, but maybe even a few more months after the birth).

People (read: you) aren't comfortable with this sort of nuance, and would prefer that you be all one way all the time. This is a big thing you're doing, and you need to feel clean about it. Square. Orderly.

Worse, like a big ol' stormy cloud, it threatens to cast a pall over even the stuff you were jazzed about, like . . . uh, all that stuff you can't even remember being excited about because you feel so bad. A baby! You're having a baby.

This is 100,000-percent normal. This happens to women who plan their babies, too, by the way, because the whole concept of having a baby is a topsy-turvy rollercoaster of feelings and fears, wrapped into one large gestating ball of upchuck. It is common, yet you're expected to be happy about it while simultaneously wondering if you will ever take a spontaneous road trip again or run quickly through a shopping mall.

Personally, I was consumed with really annoying thoughts about my childhood that I had already spent years working through. Why were they coming back? I realized, in the end, that I was becoming a mother, a transformation that had to come with the annoying but extremely important weight of thinking about the kind of mother I had, the kind of mother I wanted, and the kind of mother I would be. These growing pains are real (and also literal).

Because I had avoided this identity most of my life—I thought, *I just won't have kids, so I won't have to deal with it*—it was a shock to my system to have to do more than just think of how my mother's mothering had affected me. I now had to contend with how it would affect my mothering. My situation could happen to anyone.

When I processed my heavy grief this way, with a side of lightly salted watermelon, it made so much more sense. I realized what I was processing was fear, confusion, and uncertainty. If I had only this one example of mothering and it was lacking, how would I find my way as a good mother? I realized the answer was in the processing. I had to feel all that stuff to start fresh with a clean slate and a new outlook about my own new identity. It was heavy stuff. It went down easier when I contained it, held it outside of myself, and examined it.

Rest assured, there *is* a somewhat healthy way to deal with this sudden emotional inventory without alienating everyone in your life. A few dos and don'ts:

DON'T Expect Anyone to Care

Okay, I don't mean this as cynically as it sounds. What I mean is, don't expect anyone you know to understand, per se, in a way that's going to make you feel better. Pregnancy, planned or not, often comes with blobby, emotional goo residue that gets on everything and simply makes no sense to the nonhijacked person with a regular, non-goo brain. (Even women I knew who had been pregnant before were a bit at a loss when presented with my goo problem—how's that for mommy amnesia.) To them, you just look like a blubbering, goo-brained whale. What's with the shame spiral, they think? Aren't you supposed to be happy and stuff?

You know how paleontologists used to think a stegosaurus had a second brain that controlled its hindquarters? It's like that with you, with a second brain controlling the hindquarters of your goo feelings. It's not very good at it, and it makes you feel heavy with the weight of the entire world's feelings. Feelings Mountain. You're climbing it.

So, when you try to tell someone that you are consumed with how heinous it felt to be thirteen, when your mom totally overreacted and sent you to that group therapy because you stole that money, and everyone treated you like a criminal, but really *they* were the criminals? Yeah, no one gets that, and moreover, you stole money once? The fuck? **DON'T** even.

DO Cry, Like, Whenever You Want

. . . in private. There are always a million reasons to cry. And when you are pregnant, there are a million and one. When you are pregnant unexpectedly, there are a billion reasons. However, if you can't control it, cry wherever you feel like it. There is almost never any other time in your life, barring the occurrence of actual tragedy, when you can cry freely and people will make some kind of space for you to blubber that doesn't come with the usual sins-of-being-a-lady firing squad.

DO Cash in on All the Obvious Pregnant Sympathies

"But I don't want to cash in on all the obvious pregnant sympathies"— YES, YOU DO. If not now, when? Being overly emotional, overly tired, or overly emotional and overly tired—now is the time for all this excess. DO wallow in it. Just do it alone or with someone who has already seen your worst side, like, whichever friend knew you when you had adult braces, or got mono.

And **DON'T** forget, you don't even need a reason for all this emotion, except you totally have one.

DO NOT Fish for Emotional Support on Social Media

That means DON'T go on Facebook and post weird, passive-aggressive, sadpants status updates like "Another day blighted by the realization that NO ONE GETS ME." Ugh, there is someone who gets you—you. Never underestimate the value of understanding yourself. I repeat, do not whine on social media, unless you are into leaving a digital record that you are a LOSER. If someone is online at 8:00 P.M. on a Friday night when you want to talk about how it felt when your mother dropped you off at the skating rink from 5:00 to 11:00 P.M. every Friday and Saturday night for five years so she could date complete weirdoes, she doesn't want to talk about it. Don't be surprised when she says, "Sux, dude. Hey, I gotta head to two-for-ones. Feel better," and then hightails it to the two-for-ones . . . in her own fridge.

DO Hang Out with Other Pregnant Women

Wherever you can find them. Form your own little support group of Blubbery Emotional Goo Sufferers or BEGS. They exist. They are all around you. Put an ad in the paper or start an ANONYMOUS Facebook group for people who feel inexplicably (or hell, explicably) bad about being pregnant but who in fact are totally more together than they realize. Like you are. These fellow sufferers will tell you many things that will reassure you: You will love being a mother. You will hate being a mother. You will still be you. You will be a totally new person. You can totally go back home again. It has been demolished, flipped, and your bedroom is now filled with stuffed animals and tiny socks. But whatever. The thing is: A baby is going to change it all, and yet, in some ways you are actually going to be more focused, more motivated, more clear about what to do with the time you have.

DO Eat Whenever the Urge Strikes

No, I am not encouraging you to overeat or recklessly disregard safe limits of weight gain (see the previous chapter). I am, however, asking you to consider the ways in which food can comfort some of these erratic, odd pangs of longing or regret or guilt or sadness that no person is equipped for.

They feel so real, these feelings, and they are, but they are nothing compared to a plate of cheese cubes, Triscuits, pepperoni slices, and freshly sliced tomatoes with a sprinkling of sea salt. Cucumbers, too? Why not! Make it a mix of tiny amounts of things you probably shouldn't eat and bigger portions of stuff you should. In other words, about the same ratio of the real, lasting feelings you are having versus the crazy ones.

DO Take the Feelings Seriously—Sorta

Don't repress anything. Talk to a doctor if you are feeling hella crazy, and he will likely tell you that the feelings are normal and temporary, because they are, but may direct you to further professional help if needed. Talk to a doctor even if you're just feeling sorta crazy. Make a list of all the stuff you're afraid of, and take it apart one by one. You will find that many of the fears are unfounded, or at least not any different from the fears you might have about driving a car or moving to Europe or any number of perfectly risky things you do all the time, or at least want to do.

> **"Everything grows rounder and wider and weirder, and I sit here in the middle of it all and wonder who in the world you will turn out to be."**
>
> —Carrie Fisher

But **DO** have a good sense of humor about it. "I'll just be over here blubbering about my childhood," was a normal refrain I made. In my head.

Do Walk

One thing really did help: walking. Sounds simple, and it is: Walk. I realized the time I felt the best was when I was moving around. It kept all the weird, bad feelings at bay, not because I was ignoring them but because I was exorcising and exercising them. Also, sunshine, hello. Take it. Wrap it around you. The world goes on.

In a way, these feelings were useful. But they also had a mind of their own—like that stegosaurus brain. And I was way too tired to constantly combat it. That second brain was not a fun friend, but it was the kind of friend who gives you a tough talking to when you need it.

DO Be Nice to Yourself

It's really important while you're carrying around this deal-with-your-shit brain that you gently settle into the crazy of it all. I know, this is kind of the theme of this book, and who knew pregnancy would involve so much settling? Be kind to yourself.

Let's call it *sitting* instead. Sit into the crazy. Plop thy hind end down onto the soft pillow of crazy. It sounds, er, crazy, but if it helps, and you find the experience of pregnancy to be a bit claustrophobic, it's not entirely insane to think of pregnancy as a jail term, because it kind of is. You're physically isolated, your movements are severely limited, and your ass is no longer your own. But the sentence ends with one sweet, high-action prison break, and believe me, the sun shines even warmer when you haven't seen it in ages.

STAGE **3**:

LOGISTICS

• • •

REAL-LIFE STUFF TO FIGURE OUT

15.

WHAT WILL AN UNPLANNED BABY DO TO MY RELATIONSHIP?

The question is not *what* will the baby do, but *when* will it do it. In other words, there's no doubt having a baby will do something to your relationship—it's virtually impossible that it won't change it. A baby changes pretty much all your relationships—those with other humans, pets, and yourself. But whether that change will be good, bad, or crazy is up in the air. It mostly depends on what kind of relationship you've got. Given that this pregnancy was unplanned, you might have some extra wrenches thrown in. Just for fun.

For instance:

If Your Relationship Is Super Solid

This seems ideal, right? A relationship with a proven ability to survive already under its belt is a great foundation for having a baby, even if you didn't plan it. Take comfort in knowing you've worked through issues, faced some fears, resolved conflict, and genuinely like each other.

Warning: Just don't get too cavalier. Sure, you got it good. Do you still "got it good" after three nights of no sleep in a row with a colicky infant? Are you cuddly with a case of mastitis? What happens if you don't want to have sex during the ENTIRE PREGNANCY (and then for six months after)? Hardcore logistical changes, like the lack of free time, the physical and emotional difficulties of pregnancy, and difficulty socializing or keeping up a gym routine in those early weeks and months can make people grouchier than a cafeteria lady on fish-stick day.

Whatever you do, don't take for granted what you've got, because you will encounter entirely new kinds of conflicts and new levels of negotiating. Babies can disrupt otherwise great relationships by taking away the very spontaneity and free time that might have made them so great in the first place. They can also bring warmth and joy and spontaneity into your life in a way you actually didn't think was possible.

Protip: Spend the next nine months talking this shit out like crazy, and keep it real honest. What are your biggest fears? Who will do what? What is an ideal scenario for work schedules, daycare, weekends, free time, hobbies, etc.? No, you can't predict exactly what your baby's needs will be, or hell, even what your own will be after it's all said and done. But you have to start the conversation now about what you picture it being like, and strategies for how you'll adjust.

If Your Relationship Is Pretty Good

You've resolved some conflict, but you have issues like anyone. You're happy, but you've got sore spots that keep coming up and don't seem to get resolved. No need to declare your relationship a disaster zone just yet. Nonetheless, you should be pretty cognizant of these weak spots, because a baby is going to magnify them like a giant, ant-burning, er, magnifying glass.

Warning: If you don't get enough free time as it is, you might go nuts when you're stuck with the baby all weekend for a teething spell and you're nursing. If your partner already feels like he does more cleaning than you, he might get really resentful when he's doing double the laundry and dishes (for cloth diapers and bottle sanitizing) while you lie on the couch and moan. Whatever seems slightly unequal about your deal might suddenly become enormous.

Protip: Don't lose sight of why you're together in the first place, and keep working on the issues. Consider getting some counseling while you are pregnant to come up with a roadmap of how you'll deal with things when they flare up. Try thinking of these flare-ups the way you would treat a rash. Identify them, put some salve on them, and at least agree to give them some breathing room while you avoid crazy emotional fights. (Easier said than done!) It's important to realize that no one has a perfect relationship. You might find that in many ways, the baby makes the priorities super clear, and you're able to let go of a lot of stuff you thought mattered, because neither one of you has the time, or the energy, to actually care about it anymore.

> **"Parenthood is the passing of a baton, followed by a lifelong disagreement as to who dropped it."**
>
> —Robert Brault

If You're Totally Casual

If you got knocked up by someone who is your hookup bud, your casual fling, a one-night stand, an insta-dude, then it's impossible to say what happens next. Was he a good guy? A complete douche? A scammer? Maybe you want the relationship to move to the next level.

The problem is, in this case, that's the equivalent of meeting a dude today and going to senior prom with him tomorrow.

Warning: There's the movie *Knocked Up*, where the most inexplicable pairing turns completely stable but not without a few pretty great meltdowns along the way. Life is not a movie, but hey, it could happen. While it's certainly possible your casual fling could pull a Seth Rogen, read the baby books, ditch the bong, and become a totally stand-up dude, what are the odds? Don't eliminate the possibility, but plan for reality.

Protip: Consider the co-parenting movement, where two people who both want to procreate but cannot stand the thought of actually cuddling on a couch together have a baby together and save money to send it to great schools. Sure, you did it hella out of order, but this doesn't mean you can't approach this thing like a business arrangement, and with civility. If that seems insane to your booty call, give it time and distance, and try again. Keep your expectations realistic.

If the Relationship Is Nutso Toxic

At least you'll know where your baby gets it from? I kid. A nutso relationship is no joke, and no baby should be exposed to that. You don't need psych studies to tell you that your job is to create both an emotionally and physically stable environment for your baby. Parents fail to do this all the time, and never forget: this is how really juicy memoirs get written that get turned into motion pictures.

Warning: Do not waste time wishing the relationship were better. Deal with the relationship as it is, and take a good, hard, objective look at it. Talk it over out loud with someone really astute if you feel confused. List pros and cons to parenting with this person, and make a decision that's best for you and your baby, not just your rent or your pride. Can it be saved? Can it be improved? Can you get it, at least, to a functioning co-parenting state?

Protip: Counseling is a must, and you need to get this relationship figured out and on track or out of your life. Whatever you do, don't spend nine months mired in dysfunction with an unsuitable partner while you're growing a baby. If it's time to break out, do it fast and do it clean.

If You Wanted a Baby but the Other Person Did Not

Is this your consolation-prize baby? You don't want a consolation-prize baby. You want a partner who is super excited or at least eventually (and quickly) comes around to this whole baby thing. It will be difficult to go through all the hard parts if the other person is always like, "SEE?! TOLD YOU!"

Warning: This is potentially the hardest scenario of all, because you really need to be surrounded by a supportive partner. It is just so critical. Can you do this thing without that? Yeah, you could do it without your elbow, but do you want to?

Protip: Get thee to a counselor. Get your partner to lay the truth on the table. Get your partner to talk real talk about what he or she is willing to do here. Respect the person's wishes, which is to say that you gotta do what you gotta do and cut your losses and get your life together now.

. . .

Ultimately, no matter what kind of relationship you bring a surprise baby into, there are some tried-and-true tips for dealing with your baby daddy that will help either way, such as:

» **Ask for What You Want:** This sounds easy enough—talk about what you want (even if you're not together with your baby daddy romantically!). But that kind of openness requires both people to know what they want and say what they want. If you have issues doing this already, pregnancy will not make it any easier. Do you need to sleep late on Saturdays? Can your husband sleep late on

Sundays? Do you need help with the diapers but want to be left alone for feedings? Say it.

» **Attempt Democratic Baby-Raising:** When it comes to having a baby, splitting the duties democratically may not mean equally. Case in point: My husband would love nothing more than to hold the baby while she cries, but my daughter decided early on that when she's upset, she wants Mommy and Mommy is moi. Because I am still the go-to person for boo-boos and night terrors, I'm doing a shit ton of emotional baby work whether I have the free hands or not. The solution? My husband cooks. We just agreed this made sense. I grab the baby most times she cries, and he cooks. Please note that we could not, by the way, have ever, ever devised this plan before she was born.

» **Keep Compromising:** A compromise with a baby might mean that you go out with your friends every Friday night but he gets to play guitar for one hour each night at home. It's what you make it. The key, again, is that you work from an open, honest playing field where you lay on the table what you actually want. Otherwise, how can you ever get it?

» **Keep Communicating:** While this usually means talking about your feelings, dreams, and wishes—and I'm certainly in agreement that you should be able to do this—I'm also talking about the ability to communicate logistics. Baby logistics. If one of you is a talker and the other is the wordless type and you both intend to raise this child together, there will be confusion.

When you have a kid, everything needs to be hashed out—the picking up, the putting down, who handles bedtime, naps, bottles, breasts (okay, the person with the breasts handles the breasts, and also the baby will handle them beyond all comprehension). It might seem obvious, but if you are sitting there nursing a child, wishing you had a glass of water, don't think you can convey that to your husband telepathically. Not even if you're mad because he is enjoying what seems like the greatest luxury in the universe, lying on the couch without a tiny person attached to him, looking at his iPhone. Nope, try again. Ask. Out loud. With words.

» **Keep Laughing:** If those farts—yours, his, or the baby's—aren't funny at this point, you're fucked. Sorry.

» **Keep Trying:** Whatever is bothering one of you has got to get sorted out, and that means go over the issue like you're a detective on a cold case. Maybe there's a hot lead you missed, a clue you underestimated. Reframe the debate, get outside of your own head, and take this thing down. Treat it like a science problem, and try to detach emotionally as much as humanly, hormonally possible, which is not very much but is still doable. The key here is that both parties have to want to solve shit. But nothing is worse than unspoken resentment + diaper blowouts. It just sucks.

» **Really Make Time for Each Other:** It sounds cheesy, because it kinda is, but it matters. The time you make for each other does not have to double as a greeting card, or a Valentine's-style date night, or be the equivalent of a long-stemmed red rose. It's actually pretty simple: If you like watching movies, watch a movie together every once in a while, even if it's interrupted, even if you fall asleep. It really is the trying to make the time that counts. Make your partner a favorite meal or buy him a cool shirt. It's little shit that makes people remember that you are remembering them. Babies are tiny, hands-on, needy balls. They take it all. Remember to give something to your partner, too.

» **Keep Talking:** Negotiating, compromising, childrearing, loving—it all takes a fuckload of words. So keep using them. It's an ongoing conversation, this whole crazy mess. If you can't keep talking, then at least start signing. Hell, text if you have to. God knows there will be many times when you need someone to walk over and scratch your ass but can't risk waking the baby.

If Your Dude Doesn't Like Talking

All of this advice centers around one thing: communication with your partner. Contrary to popular opinions, dudes actually talk just as much, if not more, than women do. It's feelings in particular they aren't as equipped to reel off even while sleeping, the way women can. Thanks, cultural conditioning.

But if you're having trouble getting a dude to communicate, you're going to have to learn his language. If he can't openly express his feelings, perhaps he can leave clues about his needs, wishes, and limitations. Can he make you a PowerPoint presentation? Write a rap song? Perform an interpretive dance? Create an animated short expressing his need for three hours a week to himself? This shit matters. Whatever it takes, just get the nugget of truth out of him about where he's willing to meet you, and where he needs to be met. When language fails you, create your own.

16.

WORKING WHILST PREGNANT

Oh, but about your job. You will need to keep showing up and caring. It's true.

Here's the thing: I actually loved my job! Yet one of the biggest disappointments I experienced while surprise-pregnant was not the heartbreaking realization that I could no longer eat hot dogs topped with raw cookie dough but, rather, that pregnancy is not the free ride on the job I'd hoped it would be. I still had to show up at work most days and actually pretend to care, in spite of the fact that literally all I could think about was how much my life felt just like an episode of literate *Teen Mom*. I was so emotionally drained by my surprise pregnancy that I had little energy left for my work. Who could blame me?

What's more, thanks to big-shot, hardworking CEOs like Marissa Mayer, pregnant women are actually doing their jobs and doing them well these days, making it all the more difficult for the rest of us who want to skate awkwardly by while we right our emotional ship. (Thanks!?)

The good news is that stereotypes about women's work ethic while gestating means expectations are now at record lows for you, so low in fact that even the tiniest amount of effort—showing up at all, for instance—is considered above and beyond the call of duty. Watch out: You could even find yourself in line for a promotion by merely doing your job. So you have a little leeway while you're dealing with first-trimester nausea. Oh, and that life-altering news that you're carrying a baby.

A BIG-FAT-EXCEPTION ALERT: There are, sadly, jobs where this type of sympathy is in short supply, such as being in the military or working someplace full of martyr-type women. The martyr-type woman is the woman who has done it all and never missed a day of work to do it. Her morning sickness was worse than yours, she had every side effect in the book, and she still arrived early and stayed late. Did I mention she was carrying triplets? She gave birth riding an escalator built entirely out of malaria and was back to work in less than an hour. Even when not pregnant, she is the sort of person who gave a company-saving PowerPoint presentation while nursing her hospitalized mother, and she can regularly be seen passing kidney stones while reorganizing the office break room.

If you work with this kind of woman, and she has any modicum of power over whether you will keep your job, you're hosed. I'm sorry. I hope like hell you saw this coming and started stockpiling cash long ago in preparation to leave this job. Screw her, but you're better off without her and any place that employs her. And no, I know what you're thinking, and now is not the time to wage war with a Queen Bee such as this. You've got a job to keep.

You might, on the other hand, find yourself loving your job even more. Your job could be a godsend, a refuge from the turmoil of this surprise pregnancy and a great way to ignore the discomfort. Some women are able to bury themselves in their work to pass the aching boredom of pregnancy, right up to the bitter end! While I'm still not sure these women are human, you could strike gold and be one of them.

If you're not one of those job-loving pregnant women, and going to work every day feels like jury duty on a tax-evasion case, you're in luck. There's still a relatively smooth road ahead if you just follow my simple rules. The irony of these rules is that they are, in fact, taken verbatim from the bible of bad employees everywhere. The key is to be the kind of bad employee who actually *looks* like a model worker in spite of her lack of a valuable contribution. I call them good-shitty employees, and I have had the distinct advantage of working with one of them. They do very little work of substantive value and are bafflingly praised at every turn. Learn from them! Beat them at their own game! Or at least join them till you push out this baby!

Rule #1: Do Your Job, or at Least Appear To

This one seems obvious—duh, do your job. If you feel like doing your job because part of you or all of you still loves it, great, awesome, lucky you, way to stay focused. Please bottle that and sell it, stat.

But the cold, hard reality is that when you are pregnant you are likely to be, on occasion, far too consumed with precisely how much your latest sonogram resembles Radiohead singer Thom Yorke, or the weirdo factoid that you've actually doubled your blood volume, to care about the company's latest logo redesign challenge. Let's face it, there is even more to think/panic about when you weren't expecting this pregnancy.

Even if you are sitting online wondering how on Earth you'll find affordable daycare for this child, you best believe you need to make it look like you are as engaged as ever. This means learning how to "look busy" and "appear to be thinking about the company," and also known as keeping one work-related document open at all times, and making important-sounding phone calls. Other tactics: Taking a long time to "catch up on e-mail" and other sundry tasks that actual workers can do relatively quickly but that good-shitty employees learn to make take a full three days out of their week. Stretch it out! Make it count! You're nothing if not thorough.

Rule #2: Meet Important Deadlines

Shitty-good employees inevitably do a few things right in the service of mediocrity: They don't miss any obvious deadlines where the blame could easily fall to them. Shared deadlines are ripe for skipping, however, and cleverly bad employees miss them constantly, leaving everyone else to scramble to cover their absence, since it's always easy to point fingers and spread blame elsewhere. It's your job to prioritize what really needs to be done and what can be "forgotten" if necessary.

Unlike them, you have a real excuse: You wouldn't believe how much pregnancy amnesia can screw up everything. But unlike them, no one wants to hear your female excuse. So keep a calendar if you have to, and check it every time you pop a fresh prenatal vitamin.

Rule #3: Never Use Your Pregnancy as a Direct Excuse

Yep. I know. It sounds crazy—wasn't I just telling you to take every bit of pregnancy sympathy you could while the gettin' was good and swollen? Indeed, I did. Wouldn't you get mucho sympathy for calling in with morning sickness? Maybe in the short term. But it must never look like you are using your newfound status to your advantage. This helps you appear *so* dedicated to the company that you would not let this pesky pregnancy interfere with your productivity.

Do not reference your pregnancy in any statement that resembles a reason for being late or remiss. You do not have morning sickness, you're simply "under the weather." You're not having early contractions, you're just a spastic robot-dancer who LOOVES your job! Let your manager make a silent note of the whys and hows, but never let it back up on you. Even if your water breaks directly onto the shoes of the CEO's nephew, who happens to be an intern, just say "Splash!" and walk off all sassy. Mic drop. Mystique.

Rule #4: Surprise Everyone with Great Ideas Now and Then

Come up with a few new ideas you've been tossing around to improve your workplace. Casually offer them just after you "forgot" a deadline or turned in a less-than-excellent report. In other words, just when people might be questioning your effort, throw out one of your gems to turn the tide of public opinion 180 degrees. Who cares if the ideas are not brilliant (don't make them suck *too* badly, though) or are not realistic anytime soon (don't suggest everyone relocate to the moon)—just come up with some decent, reasonably possible ideas. Hell, some of them can even be real ones. And if you can't think of any fake ones? Repurpose old ones! Last month you suggested an office-wide suggestion box. This month? An office-wide IDEA box. Totally different. If anyone mentions it, feign a vague amnesia attributed to this sweltering day, or that frosty front moving in.

Rule #5: Disagree Thoughtfully

In group meetings where ideas are bandied about, try taking issue with something—anything—at least a little. While you risk looking like a naysayer, it at least makes it look like you are engaged and actually paying attention in the meeting. Just don't disagree so much that you find yourself with any extra responsibilities or are labeled office crank. That title only works for men, and those men get promoted. Women will find themselves labeled "emotional." Extra credit: disagree with a joke or a wink.

Rule #6: Become Indispensible at Something

Since you probably want to return to your job (or perhaps arrange a mom-friendly schedule) post-baby, it's time to "own" something of importance at work. Something no one else can do. Maybe it's becoming BFFs with your top client. Maybe it's charming the IT guy to fix the server in a timely manner. Maybe it's keeping the coffee stocked. Whatever it is, be known as THE person who can do that task. Imagine the chaos that will ensure when you're on maternity leave! The company will be *begging* you to return to work in some fashion. And *you'll* have the upper hand in those negotiations.

Rule #7: Fill Your Plate with Easy-for-You Tasks

The beauty of this rule is knowing which tasks will *seem* complicated or tedious to the higher-ups, but which are, in fact, a breeze for you. Try delivering everyone's mail in person around the office without being asked—a job most people find tedious but a slowed-down worker such as yourself could perform with ease. If your bosses are old and intimidated by the Big Scary Worldwide Web, you could be a real asset on the team by simply running the company Twitter account and refashioning yourself as a "social media maven." Whatever they are, take on tasks that require zero intellectual output on your part. That way, you have free time to compare baby bumps with Beyonce and consider nursery paint colors.

Rule #8: Make Cookies—A LOT

Everyone loves cookies. Everyone loves people who bring cookies. No one can be mad at the person who brought the cookies. No one can especially be mad at the pregnant lady who brought the cookies, so long as she does not eat them (all).

Bring the cookies. This helps if, despite your best efforts, a handful of smarter, more intuitive colleagues are on to you.

Rule #9: Act as if You Are Coming Back, but Plan as if You Are Not

Finally, you must prep for your potential exit, or at least your maternity leave. Document your work responsibilities and plan for a successor. This successor might just be filling in for your maternity leave, or could be taking over forever if you never intend to step foot in that godforsaken hellhole again. Making a "leave plan" allows you to both look like a loyal worker and prepare for a smooth exit should you get the fuck out of Dodge. (P.S. Also be super extra nice and friendly to your temporary successor, because you do not want to give that person a reason to hate/upstage/outperform you.)

Even if you really are planning to keep your job, realize that in spite of the legal protections you think you have or ought to have while pregnant, there are all kinds of loopholes that businesses can use to fire you while pregnant or on leave, and they are perfectly within their right to do so. It happens all the time, and it is insane. Even if your company seems great, you gotta look out for number one now.

Even if you totally plan on coming back to work after you have the baby and tell everyone earnestly that you really actually totally are, no one thinks that you actually mean it. Regardless, never so much as wink-wink/nudge-nudge to ANYONE you work with, not even your best friend, that you are not coming back post-baby. It could actually really jeopardize things like maternity leave pay, a.k.a. worker's comp.

Rule #10: Live on the Edge of TMI

If you need to leave early one day for a "doctor's appointment" (a.k.a. addressing a cupcake craving), give your boss just a taste of your medical issues. Start to say something about your "pelvic floor," "gastrointestinal distress," or "hot yeast infection," and your boss will send you out the door faster than you can say "Flagyl." NO ONE wants to hear ANYTHING about a pregnant woman's body. Throw out a few key words and you'll get whatever you need.

As you sail or slog through the rest of your pregnancy, use what is left of your energy to focus on rebuilding your cubicle out of smoke, mirrors, and mediocrity. Be the best little weakest link you can be. It's the only way to survive.

17.

FIGURING OUT YOUR MATERNITY LEAVE

Maternity leave in the United States is a hilarious, mostly fictional thing, and if you never realized you were supposed to be angry about this before, you will definitely want to take a minute to get good and steamingly angry about it now. The United States. is still the only western country with zero paid leave as policy. There are 163 other countries that pay women to take MANDATORY LEAVE! Are you a feminist? Become a feminist! Or at least just get pissed.

How is anyone supposed to have babies when even the government won't make your employer give you a few measly paid weeks off to take care of the thing? What are you, some baby-having superwoman who's supposed to give birth mid-Excel spreadsheets? And how, pray tell, should you pay for said birth when you're not getting paid? How can the world even work like this? Okay, done? Okay.

Now, there is something called the Family Medical Leave Act (FMLA), which gives you up to twelve weeks of UNPAID time to chill with a new baby without fear of losing your job. The problem is that FMLA comes with some very sneaky caveats. One, this law only applies to companies with over fifty employees. Two, those companies can sidestep this particular leave thing-a-ma-what if they can argue that your position can't be vacated for that amount of time because it's too critical to the operation.

So here's where you cross your fingers and hope your job is just important enough to matter but not so important as to get you fired. And pregnant women can totally be fired. Wait, but isn't that against the law? Nope. You're thinking of the law where they can't be discriminated against. They can be fired. There is no pregnancy job-firing immunity lotion like that stuff they give you to prevent stretch marks, which also doesn't work, BTW.

But! Some companies do offer paid leave straight out of their pockets and into yours. I do not know what those companies are, or if they only exist in San Francisco, or if you have to be born into a secret order of elite women to have one of those jobs. I just know that no one I have ever known has had one of those jobs.

What a lot of companies offer as "paid leave" is really disability insurance or worker's compensation, and pregnancy falls under this umbrella. Try to ignore the initial cognitive dissonance of having to accept that procreating is legally a handicap for the purposes of this program, especially because by the end of the third trimester you will agree that it is. This is insurance. It is partial wage compensation. Sometimes it's a benefit you get automatically that your employer covers. Sometimes it's offered to you as a benefit you can pay a few dollars a month for.

P.S. The disability payment is not disbursed until the baby is officially outside of you, so even if you go on bed rest for the last six weeks, no worker's comp in your paws until the little one arrives. Not almost arrives, not "is on the way," not "the baby called and she'll be here next week, honest," but actually arrived.

The catch here, and there is always a catch, is that you typically have to have been paying into this program (or your company has to have been paying in for you) BEFORE you got knocked up for you to be able to draw from it. So if you are feeling pretty bad about the fact that back on sign-up day, you were too young and virile and not gonna need it to pay a few dollars, I am very, very, personally sorry. It coulda helped.

I personally worked for a nice company that paid this disability coverage in full for employees as a benefit. But right after I found out I was pregnant, the company I worked for was sold. The new company wanted to honor the old benefits, but some of them, like disability coverage, would now be partly covered by employees. Suddenly, even though I was signing up for the new coverage, I was technically coming into the new job as pregnant, so I had not been "paying in" to my new employer's plan and was initially denied coverage. Luckily, being pregnant and hormonal meant that it took exactly zero effort to be a huge bitch about it, the good kind of bitch who gets shit done. I was begrudgingly covered as if I'd been paying in all along. (Because I had been!) Be a good bitch who gets shit done if you need to. This is your life and your baby's life, not an etiquette pageant.

But if you don't have this money or a paid leave option, there is still hope. You can try what many women are forced to do and combine all forms of sick days, paid time off, unpaid time off, and vacation time to create a kind of patchwork of time off for at least a few weeks post-baby. The key here is to use as little time off as you can during the pregnancy so you have max time on the back end.

You are correct, this sounds truly impossible given all the doctor checkups, fatigue, and various ailments that will leave you needing more days off than an aspiring actor at a restaurant gig. But trust me, you would much rather have the time off after the baby than before. Schedule doctor's visits before or after work, or fit them in on lunch breaks. Work from home if it's at all possible on days you are feeling sluggish. Hire your double to go to work and pretend to be you while you get checkups. Do whatever it takes to conserve what time off you have to recover without forcing yourself to do the worst thing in the universe: care about an office job while you are trying to heal your vagina. (Of course, if you have a job you love and want to work throughout the labor itself, go, produce, succeed, give birth mid-Excel spreadsheets! I applaud you.)

The other aspect of your maternity leave to figure out is what you'll do after it's over, assuming you plan to return to work. The one key thing to making this work is being super upfront with your employer about what you're aiming to do. Planning this in advance (along with a well-considered strategy about what will get handled in your absence) is a huge asset here. Perhaps there's some aspect of your work you're happy to continue to oversee, and can get paid a partial salary for. Perhaps you can swing child care a few days a week, and that's enough time to come in with laser-like focus and knock it out.

If you're in good standing, your boss won't want to lose you and may be willing to work with you on a completely new schedule, or give you a more manageable re-entry back into work by only pulling a part-time shift for the first few months back.

18.

FINDING GOOD CHILD CARE

You have been busting a hump to prepare for welcoming a baby into your life, but if you plan on going back to work, suddenly you have to reconcile handing your bundle over to someone else. While this sounds like a great excuse for more cognitive dissonance–inspired pregnancy eating, rest assured there's no time for that. Yes, you actually have to start planning this now, before the baby arrives! Most likely, the problem won't be finding child care, it will be finding *good* child care.

The good news: Citizens of the world feel like crucial participants in the business of raising a good citizen, and everyone wants to join this welcome wagon. The bad news: How the hell are you supposed to know which of these Mary Poppins you can trust?

Luckily, the same cynicism that made you not want a baby in the first place comes in extra handy here. If you know your own weaknesses in the kid-friendly department, it's easier to imagine what the ideal caregiver should possess—in spades—to earn the right to watch your child, and all for the low cost of one month's rent, two if you live anywhere that isn't New York or Los Angeles. That's right. You will pay anywhere from, oh, $600 to upwards of $1,200–$2,000 a month. This is, no question, the biggest expense of having a kid in the early years (unless you are the mother of budding fashionista Suri Cruise).

Here are some basic options:

» Family, if they are not crazy, drunk hyenas.
» A nanny is another great choice but a huge luxury, very expensive, and only one person, a person who will call in sick and take a vacation and should be paid a fair, living wage. With benefits.
» A daycare is at least a reliable, socializing institution where you can drop a kid off for a full workday. Sure, it's crazy expensive, but sometimes the fee covers diapers, lunch, and snacks. Sometimes it doesn't.

By the time your maternity leave starts, which could be weeks or months or literally minutes after you give birth, you'll need to have already started thinking somewhere in the foggy depths of your brain about how you want this whole child care thing to play out.

If you haven't yet, no worries! Some coworker with a three-year-old will helpfully remind you any second now by casually mentioning that you were supposed to get on the good preschool lists six months before birth. Some of them have waiting lists!

"Um, do you mean daycare?" you'll ask with hilarious naiveté.

Did you know that daycare is called preschool? Even when it's just daycare?

Daycare is a place that watches your kid and changes her diapers and does lots of art projects.

Preschool is a place that watches your kid and changes her diapers and does lots of art projects once she turns three years old and lists the name of an Italian person who lived a long time ago on its website.

Kidding—your kid should definitely be potty trained by three if you want her to go to a good preschool. And sometimes the person in the bio is German.

If all this sounds needlessly anxiety-inducing, that's because it is. Somewhere between freaking the fuck out and not giving a shit is the correct way to feel. The problem is that reaching this nirvana of caring but not caring is apparently a lifelong process, and you've only got a few weeks.

Since this pregnancy was unexpected, I'm guessing that you weren't on a waiting list the day after you peed on that stick. It's okay: the waiting list thing is real, but daycares have the occasional open spot when a kid moves, leaves, ages out, etc., and you can often get around waiting lists. So don't panic.

Perhaps one of the reasons you didn't expect this pregnancy is because you weren't sure that you'd be a good parent. This is good, because it means you have actual standards, standards so high you were willing to eliminate yourself from the running of parenting. Think of the number of people who had children without a thought in the world as to their capacity for raising them. Let's put that knack for baseless judgment to good use when you vet these crazy gargoyles to see if they can care for your precious children with the kind of standards only people like us who weren't sure we wanted kids can really understand. Here's what you should consider.

Ask Around

Everyone looks like a paragon of pristine care on the Internet, so the best way to find a good daycare is to ask other parents where they send their kids. Parents whose judgment you trust, of course. At the very least, these recommendations can give you a place to start so you're not fumbling around with a list of fifty places to check out.

Know Your Own Comfort Zone

Every parent is different, so note your own comfort zone: one parent's version of a sweet old grandma daycare director is another's untrained bag of bones who's going to accidentally feed her child her heart palpitations medication while simultaneously falling and breaking her hip.

You Get What You Pay For

A daycare is a business, okay? There are shitty ones and excellent ones, and even the excellent ones can fall short of the glory, simply because they are not you. We searched daycares for months in Los Angeles and found that the cheaper the daycare, the closer to the freeway, the more likely the food wasn't organic, the more likely some random guy named Bob was part of the operation.

If it was stupid-cheap affordable, there was a hot curling iron left on in the bathroom, the one with the door wide open with kids running in and out of it. If it was expensive, it was really expensive, as in $30K a year up front, but was conveniently advertised as the first step on the way to Harvard. We bit the bullet and shot for the middle, paying more than we'd budgeted at first, figuring it would burn a lot more to be broke with a kid almost in Harvard than broke with a kid with a curling iron burn.

Homegrown Can Be Homey—or Horrific

Home daycare centers can be great because they are often smaller and more comfortable, and feel safer. When done well, they are run by lovely people who have wonderful, idyllic homes that you wish you could live in. Sometimes they can cut you a deal on a deposit, or work with you when you're strapped for a month's dues, because they are much more personal about the care. They might also be more flexible on scheduling and pickup and dropoff times.

But when done poorly, the daycare provider might cut some corners, by letting her husband, the one you've never really talked to because he seems to mutter and act kinda surly, watch your kid when she has a doctor's appointment without even telling you. Not okay.

Education/Experience

No, you don't need a master's degree to love a child or care for it well. You do need a master's to certify in early childhood education. It's not a deal-breaker if the person doesn't have a master's, because tons of experience can make up for this. So preferably the director of the daycare you're about to pay two car payments has read more books than you on this subject, cared for dozens of children for more than a decade, and won't be "winging it" like you are.

First Aid

Anyone who cares for your child should be able to perform CPR. End of story. Can you do it? Doesn't matter. (Well, you should be able to do it, of course.) What you have that the average stranger/daycare provider does not is the motivation to learn to fly on command, if necessary, to remove your child from danger or into an ER, should that horrible, unthinkable, but all-too-common situation arise. Short of that, every other caregiver entrusted with your child must be a paragon of up-to-date CPR cards.

"Well, now, that's a funny story," should never be the first sentence uttered by a potential caregiver when you ask if she is certified.

Good Location

I don't mean the Beverly Hills of daycares; I merely mean that when you drive to drop off your kid at someone else's joint for eight hours, it shouldn't make you weep with despair, fear for your life, or experience a strange, sinking sensation.

This means: Do not send your child to daycare next to the freeway if you can help it, or next to the industrial waste center, or next to the nuclear plant. Will she probably be fine hanging out there if the center is otherwise a solid place? Sure? I guess? If it's not for that long? Just think: You've got the rest of your life to play roulette with educational choices; don't sweat the first crucial years of your child's life with a shoddy daycare. Make it your top priority.

Something else to consider is how convenient the location is. Is it on your way to work, or 25 miles in the opposite direction? Is it in between both parents' daytime locations? Is it close to your office, so you can pop in at lunch once in a while?

Bells and Whistles

Don't make the mistake of believing you have to pay more for organic mangoes and yoga classes, unless you live somewhere that doesn't offer that traditionally. In Los Angeles, even the shittiest daycare has your kid doing downward facing dog every now and then. What you want is a philosophy of care that matches your own. Don't have one yet? Read on.

Philosophy of Care

Will your kid be an artistic type or more of a logical thinker? The good news is that until that kid is three or four, it's not like it matters in terms of care. Mostly what he needs to thrive is the same: a warm, loving, engaging environment where he doesn't get hit in the face by an eight-year-old with anger issues. Early on, you just want an attentive caregiver—someone who seems naturally suited to children, genuinely warm, and talks freely with you about discipline and direction for your child. Later on, you might go in a more free-spirited or science-brainy direction for your kid.

No need to figure that out now, especially since you actually can't. Or at least I've never met a baby I could predict would rather count than paint, but perhaps everyone else knows something I don't. Wouldn't be the first time.

Transparency

If they don't issue a written incident report for every significant boo-boo (and there should not be lots of these), then the daycare is doing it wrong. If the daycare wants you to warn them before you stop by, the daycare is doing it wrong. If the daycare lets anyone you haven't been introduced to and given credentials for step in and care for the children in their absence, they are doing it wrong. If the daycare suddenly decides to change locations and doesn't mention the new location until they are already all moved in and it's too late to change it and the new location happens to be 5 feet from one of the busiest freeways in the entire country and they are real defensive about it when you mention it, run, don't walk, to the nearest onramp. And then detail all this for Yelp the second you get home.

Vibes

Yes, it sounds hokey and spiritual and it's not scientific at all, but ultimately, regardless of experience and education and facilities, the people you trust to care for your kid should make you feel totally, completely comfortable. If there's any weirdness at all, bail. It doesn't matter if you can't identify what it is. If they tend to be unable to explain injuries or there are lots of injuries or you just don't like the way the husband is always hanging around acting moody, get out. Underneath the fog, sleeplessness, and grouchiness of your new-mother brain are some instincts. They feel judgy and suspicious because they are supposed to be. Trust them.

19.

YOU ARE ABOUT TO LOSE ONE PRECIOUS COMMODITY FOREVER: FREE TIME

Before you get too far down Pregnancy Road: There's a lot of advice out there about things you, as a woman, should experience last-hurrah-style before you have your first baby: go to Burning Man, join a cult, take peyote in the desert—okay, maybe those are all the same thing. But there's not much advice on what you can do quickly to sow those wildly bloated oats if you're already knocked up and didn't get a chance beforehand to live it up like Tila Tequila on spring break. (If this isn't your first baby, see the next chapter.)

I'm sure you could, while pregnant, still go to shows and bars and parties and things where people drink and laugh, and try to pretend you are Tila Tequila on spring break drinking O'Doul's or whatever. I read about these women, who assert "I'm pregnant, not dead!" and I commend their pregnant aliveness. Hat tip to you, m'lady.

But if you're like me and require some form of alcohol to hang out with strangers for more than forty minutes, this is just not viable while pregnant. Also, as previously noted, my lifestyle wasn't exactly baby-friendly. Hanging around a bunch of barflies was not going to strengthen my resolve to quit smoking or eat better or think about nursery room colors.

Remember, your life isn't actually ending, just changing dramatically. This is exciting, but it's murder on your feet. Believe it or not, you will, eventually, be able to escape again at night and get toasty on the sauce or see rock shows or go adventure skiing once your baby has safely exited your womb. What you may never have again is regular, old-fashioned, boring free time. Relish it now. Heed my words. Do not go gently into that good but overscheduled night!

I know, I know, it sounds extreme, but I cannot overstate it. Every time I try to tell someone that the free time you once had before breeding evaporates along with your placenta, they are almost certain I am lying or at the very least exaggerating. For the love of all that's horrifyingly holy, *I'm not.*

It's not that there is literally no free time, not even a second—though that is precisely how it feels. It's that any and all free time you have will feel so magical, so precious, so endangered, and so critical to recharging just to get you through the next twenty-three hours and forty-six minutes, that it's unlikely you will be able to ever enjoy it properly again. Every time you try to (gasp!) enjoy a free minute, you'll encounter the nagging sensation that it could always be better used doing something else. Something—dundundun—say it with me: productive.

Remember what *productive* used to be, or probably is in your current version of a life? It's something you choose to be when the get-shit-done mood strikes: cleaning the bathroom, scheduling an eye exam, buying a birthday gift before the person's birthday.

But believe me when I tell you that *productive* is the enemy of the well-rested new mother. It's true. Wherever there is a napping child, there is a mother nearby feeling guilty that she isn't using the time to clean or plan or organize or collect points for rejected applications to magnet schools she was never going to send her child to anyway (Los Angeles, amirite?). Even though everyone tells you to "sleep when the baby sleeps," rare is the mother who is able to go, "Screw it, I'm sleeping, too." (Is this, pray tell, the same mother who still goes to rock shows while pregnant?)

Even to this day—and I have a three-year-old—it is nearly impossible for me to sleep while my child takes her nap. I have done it fewer than five times in her entire life. I am overcome with the relentless pressure to have some me-time or betterment-of-her-life time, lest this be the one day the child decides to finally abandon naps forever.

I know, it sounds crazy. You're thinking, it can't be that bad, can it? Perhaps the problem is that science has still failed to come up with a foolproof way to explain to a childless person what it will really be like once this new pod-person arrives, so it's unlikely you've been sufficiently frightened about how limited your life will actually become compared to what you once knew. You're probably too busy being frightened about the correct kind of birth to have. (Hint: It's a trick question. The baby picks the type of birth, and she doesn't care who Ricki Lake is.)

Either way, you'll want to wallow in the freedom you have now, before you are forced to redefine freedom as the sixteen seconds it takes you to pee—and even those seconds are up for grabs by the time your little one can walk.

A really great invention would be a haunted-house version of new motherhood that wouldn't frighten you enough to give you a heart attack but maybe just enough to make you pee yourself a little (also good practice for your future). You would go to a place for a weekend stay where your time, sleep, and general well-being would be interrupted at random and without warning for the entire weekend to approximate life with a newborn. Lie down: ALARM goes off. Try to pee: Baby starts crying! Grab a cup of tea: LUKEWARM!

But, people, if you don't have the appropriate fear in you, you'll just keep sitting around being all pregnant and shit, not realizing what you're about to lose. I know this because when other people with kids tried to explain to me the rules of The New Frontier, I found their advice to be maddeningly, almost suspiciously vague.

"It changes everything," they would warn ominously but imprecisely, like an extremely vague one-person Greek chorus of doom, while slowly backing away from me.

"Everything?" I wondered aloud as I clomped back into their personal space, coming ever closer to their warn-y faces.

"Really? Literally everything? From the biggest, most abstract concepts to the tiniest details? Take, for instance, the fact that right now, I'm sitting right here eating these cheese cubes. Are you really saying I won't still be able to eat cheese cubes with cheesy abandon after the baby comes? I mean, come on! Exaggerate much?"

Yes, I really would talk this way. HORMONES. And, at this point in the conversation, the advice giver, ever emboldened by my defiance like some kind of coworker Newman, would simply nod her head and say, "Oh, you'll see."

I'll SEE, will I? A-HA! At least I'll still have my VISION, I thought smugly, proof not literally everything was going to be different after childbirth.

Of course, they were right, I was obnoxious, and everything was different after having a baby. It's not that they were lying or I was hardheaded (even though I totally am), it's that this, like so many other clichés of parenting, is one of those things you have to experience for yourself. Note: for the unexpecting expectant mother, it may take even longer for this realization to kick in, so powerful is your denial mechanism, but when it hits you, it may hit harder.

By the time I figured it all out, it was, alas, too late. One evening, as I hoisted myself into the shower days past my due date, I was finally hit with a sensation I could identify: As I stood there enjoying the leisurely pounding of a good shower spray against my aching lower back for what felt like an eternity (but which in reality was merely just over three minutes), I suddenly had the distinct feeling that I would never take a shower like this again. I couldn't really explain why I knew, I just did. Everything suddenly felt impending, as if I'd turned some kind of corner and hit a point of no return.

So I did what I hadn't done the whole pregnancy, when, especially toward the end, I was so anxious to get this thing out of me that I could scarcely pass the time calmly. I paused. I stood there a little bit longer, trying to just experience the sensation of being on the precipice, of knowing things would be different but not being able to pinpoint exactly how.

"The quickest way for a parent to get a child's attention is to sit down and look comfortable."

—Lane Olinghouse

Like trying to imagine your future husband when you haven't even met him, it was an odd sense of hope, excitement, and panic, like how it felt right before I graduated high school, or what it was like in my twenties to try to picture what my actual life and job would be like when I "grew up."

Two days later, my water broke. In the shower. The dam had burst. The heavens had heaved, and rushing out among the many clichés about miracles, game-changers, and precious moments were all the minutes and seconds of aimless, meandering, mundane, boring free time I would never get back. I would never want for it again in the exact same way—yesterday's nap on the couch while watching sitcom reruns is today's five minutes in the car alone in deafening silence eating a muffin—but I always regretted, just a little, not taking it in as fully as I should have before it was gone.

So I implore you, stop whatever you are doing right now, pregnant woman, and do the following things. Yes, your life is about to be enriched and uplifted in new, arguably more meaningful ways than what doing nothing used to do for you, but that doesn't make doing nothing any less awesome. In fact, rest assured that the concept of the gentle awesomeness of not having anything better to do is perhaps the only thing that will remain unchanged by breeding.

So even though there are always sock drawers to organize, emotions to wrangle, money to save, cat hair to eradicate, bottle nipples to sanitize, birthing plans to compose, and life insurance policies to comparison-shop for, do your life a favor and make sure that before the clock strikes baby, you've spent as much of your pregnancy as you can doing the following totally American Pregnancy Association–approved things:

» Stare at a wall.
» Spend a day doing absolutely nothing.
» Watch part of a movie. Rewatch the same part. Watch the entire movie.
» Call a friend and discuss the movie.
» Get into an argument with the friend about whether the boyfriend character is, in fact, as emotionally unavailable as all six of your friend's last boyfriends. Gah, what was she thinking? What were YOU thinking with your last TWELVE boyfriends, she counters?
» Hang up on your friend.
» Call her back.
» Apologize.
» Make some nachos.
» Go check the mail.
» Do a bunch of organizational stuff for yourself. Not for the baby! Wait, yes, also for the baby.
» But also: clean out your closet.
» Rearrange your socks.
» Throw out all your weird hats.
» Buy more weird hats!
» Knit a weird hat.

» Sleep.

» For the love of god, sleep.

» Sleep in late. In a weird hat.

» Take a nap.

» Go to bed early.

» Sleep for sixteen hours in a row.

» Make your room into a cave and sleep like you were hibernating for the winter or suddenly living in the ideal bedroom of a teenager.

» Sleep in a hotel.

» Catnap on the couch.

» Sleep whenever or wherever the mood strikes you (provided it is not while operating machinery of any kind).

» Take very long showers. Hot showers. Long baths. Hot baths. Lukewarm baths. Bubble baths. Mud baths. Swimming baths.

» Take ALL of the baths!

» Take a very, very long time in the bathroom. Make it count. Draw it out! Feel the listlessness. Lean into the experience of just you, alone in a room without anyone knocking on the door, doing whatever weird/dumb/gross/boring thing it is you need to do in there.

» Go to the grocery store and wander the aisles aimlessly.

» Go to an actual store and buy something. (Henceforth, Internet shopping will be your best friend.)

» Don't buy something.

» Buy something and then take it right back and return it.

» Buy it again.

» Lie on your bed (not on your back for too long, *cough*superior vena cava*cough*Google it*cough*Weird, right?*cough) and just do nothing.

» Do nothing some more, all day long for one entire day.

» Go see a movie at night.

» Go do anything at night!

- » Go to brunch (at night).
- » Sit around with friends talking for hours, uninterrupted.
- » Sit around with more friends talking for more hours.
- » Take a road trip somewhere more than thirty-eight minutes away.
- » Stop the car.
- » Get out of the car.
- » Look around.
- » Stand there, and this is important, looking up, not down, and around. (Henceforth, you will be looking down at your lovely baby.)
- » Look up some more.
- » Talk your sister's ear off on the phone that night.
- » Eat an extra dessert.
- » Laugh a bunch at dumb stuff.
- » Browse in a bookstore for ages.
- » Browse in a bookstore for all ages.
- » Browse in a bookstore for senior citizens.
- » Be marvelously, mundanely alive in the most leisurely, aimless way you can.
- » Eat at a salad bar.

Just kidding. Everyone knows they are loaded with bacteria.

20.

IF YOU'RE ADDING TO YOUR BROOD

Newsflash: This ain't your first rodeo. You've already got other kids—some of them undoubtedly on purpose. This means that for you, all the anxious excitement of pregnancy is rushing back up with a familiar, nauseating swirl.

The good news: You've been down this road before!

The bad news: Ugh, you've been down this road before.

You actually sort of know what you don't know. Gone is the ignorant bliss of the first-kid learning curve, and in its place, an intimate, achingly precise portrait of the toll sleeplessness, exhaustion, and diaper changing can take on your (relatively) figured-out existence. But even though you've been there, it can still throw you for a very exhausting loop.

A baby out of nowhere is still a baby out of nowhere, no matter how many babies you have. Yes, you already have an existence ordered around children, but children are likely not babies anymore, and taking the train back to baby station is a seismic psychological shift, even if you're reading this while simultaneously removing lice out of the head of your kindergartner. So anyone who makes you feel like it should be no bigs to toss another squirt of artificial butter on the popcorn of your life doesn't know what they're talking about—regarding babies or your life. Or popcorn, for that matter.

If you could sum up the trouble, it would probably go something like this: But you just finished INSERT MILESTONE HERE. Also known as: You just lost the baby weight. You just finished nursing. You just went back to work full-time. You just started to like the way you looked in a pair of jeans—hell, you just found a pair of jeans that actually fit. You just booked a bungee-jumping trip to Europe. You just figured out how to be an interesting conversationalist again. You and your husband just started having sex again, and you were just getting used to sleeping in until 8:15 A.M. You just got a kid into kindergarten and got your afternoons back. How can you possibly work one more in?

Apparently, with not that much difficulty. Studies show that the financial shock of a third baby, for instance, is nothing like the first, or even second baby, as shocks go. A recent United States Department of Agriculture report on the price tag of kids (about a quarter of a million dollars just to get one to eighteen, and that's without even necessarily making them cool), as reported in the *New York Times*, found that three-child families spend 22 percent less per child than those in the two-child norm.

This is likely in no small part due to the handy convenience of reusing gear, and the deep discounts for multiple kids for child care and tuition costs. Even if you already sold off all your gear a long time ago, take comfort that you have something first-time parents literally pay for in dollars: You know what you actually need to get a baby through her first year, so you're not gonna get suckered into dropping a small fortune on that potty with an iPad holder built in (on second thought, why tempt yourself? Do NOT Google).

Take all the comfort in these been-there advantages that you can get, because some of the challenges will no doubt be harder this time around. For one, you're older, so bouncing back from another pregnancy fueled by pepperoni-flavored nostalgia might be more difficult. For two, now you're going to be on the receiving end of jokes about recklessly populating the earth and, if this is your third baby, running zone defense. Inevitably, someone is also going to crack wise about the fact that surely by now you understand a thing or two about birth control. That person should be smacked in the face with a NuvaRing.

But time in the trenches trumps jackanapes here, too. And you have a few tricks up your sleeve that even the most persistent scavenger can't put a damper on. With all the usual noob worrying out of the way, you can actually just enjoy all the little surprise stuff a first-timer could hardly fathom, from first smiles to first steps, not to mention the many future sibling adventures in your not-so-distant future.

> **"Having one child makes you a parent; having two you are a referee."**
>
> —David Frost

The biggest mental challenge for you is to keep an open mind, take a deep breath, and get into a wide stance. This will help when the baby drops out quickly, as second and third children are notorious for doing. But also, it's a posture that will help you remind yourself that no two pregnancies are alike. That no two children are alike. And that bringing another kid into the mix will be joyous in old and new ways, difficult in old and new ways, and everything in between.

You may not be not hard-pressed to make a house kid-friendly in nine months, but you will still have to readjust the safety dial back to newborn-level concerns. You're not facing an urgent struggle to embrace the mental challenge of seeing yourself as a new parent, but, depending on the age of your kids, you'll have to reach way back into the way-back machine to remember what it meant to care for a newborn those first few weeks and months. And emotionally, you might need a minute to adjust to the plans you'll put on hold, and to accept the increased future costs that might change those family trips to Europe into camping out at parks.

But if there's one thing you know now, it's that things have a way of ending up better than planned, even when the path is less than obvious. And in thinking over all these questions and concerns, you have these four little helpers: perspective, experience, patience, and other kids.

Perspective

Having children already is a one-way ticket to Perspectiveville. What you now know is that things have a way of working out, and they really do. What you now know is that the things you think matter most are often of the least consequence when all is said and done. What you now know is that the money gets figured out, that you make do with what you've got, that brushing one's hair every day is overrated, and that the next few years of compromised sleep are happening to someone who already got through lack of sleep just fine once (or even twice) before. You can do it again, because you already did it once before. You see the bigger picture, or, rather, you see the picture after the one where you're tearing your hair out again trying to get the new baby to nap.

Experience

The things that throw most first-time parents for a loop is the rabbit hole of worry a first kid brings. But you've been there and done that. And you know that tar comes off a pastel pair of jeans with baby oil, and that a breastfed baby can go a couple of days without pooping and be just fine. You know that an ear infection doesn't always present with a fever, but two days of a certain pitch of crying and runny nose usually means one is on the horizon. This means you'll make judgment calls faster, and with more confidence, and this time, you will more likely be able to enjoy your newborn in all her newborn-ness instead of worrying about all the stuff you should be reading, learning, or doing to encourage her growth. That's gotta be worth its weight in breastfed baby poop, to say nothing of the time it's going to free up.

Patience

You might feel like it's as dried up as you thought your ovaries were, but in truth, you have a deep well of patience from having raised another kid or two already. Yes, you're going straight back to baby jail with this addition to your family—do not pass GO—but this isn't exactly uncharted territory here, nor is it permanent, which means the learning curve is not quite so curvy. When you feel more tired than you remembered, you'll push through, because you know it only *seems* like it drags on forever. When you discover that this baby needs half the sleep and twice the food as the last kid, you'll pull it together, because you'll realize that this could be the child that wins the Nobel Prize for Tireless Work on Important Subject.

Other Kids

The secret to any industrialized family unit is free labor, and your children are the little engines that could. What are they for? Puttin' to work. As someone who spent my youthful summers picking corn and cleaning out old sheds, now is as good a time as any to teach your children the ways of the world and enlist them in the care and feeding of a fellow human. This not only takes a load off, but it gives other children an active role in this new member's socialization into the family unit. Plus, it fosters empathy, nurturing, and all the other things you were previously too exhausted to impart. Besides, if there's one truism you've already learned, it's that the older the kid, the harder to force to repaint a basement. Act now.

21.

WHAT YOU SHOULD REALLY TAKE AWAY FROM BIRTHING CLASS

You may not have planned getting knocked up, but you can at least plan how your birth will go. JK! You have virtually no control over it. Of course, that's not what birthing classes will advertise. They seem to promise something quite hilarious in retrospect: the notion that you can choose how you will have your baby, and that it will actually work out that way. That if you just master a technique you will have some kind of control over what happens in that room. Ha, good one, birthing classes.

Do you want a partner to "coach" you through the process? Do you want to meditate to transcend the pain? Do you want to huff and puff your way through labor, or have the maximum freedom to move around and change positions? How the hell would you know?

You wouldn't. And even if you did know, you can't control it anyway. That's why birthing classes are such a rip-off and I can tell you everything you need to know right here. But that said, you should totally take a birthing class! Birthing classes are still important and useful, just not necessarily the way you think.

Whether HypnoBirthing, Bradley, Lamaze, or Alexander, all of them are ultimately selling you the same thing: a series of possible ways your birth could go, and a series of possible tools you could use if your birth happens to go the way that lots of births do go. You could read this in a book or online. What you can't get in a book or online is the delivery method: a convenient, therapy-like meeting where you can learn nearly every possible way a pregnant woman can look, feel, talk, and think. Basically, it's an outlet to be your blobby, goo-brained self among other blobby goo-brains. It's truly an eye-opener because of how much it normalizes the pregnancy experience, and that alone is worth the price of admission. Anything that gives you a chance to go somewhere and relax, learn, open up, and blow off steam is worth its weight in lanolin.

And yes, you will learn a lot, including things like: what's happening to your body, how labor feels when it starts, what false labor is, how an ideal birth should go, how there's no such thing as an ideal birth, hospitals versus home births, and how best to work as a team with your partner. Tools imparted include techniques that can ease pain, help breathing, aid relaxation, and deal with medical personnel.

But what you should *actually* take away from birthing classes is the following:

Your Labor Will Go Fine, Unless It Doesn't

Everything will likely go off totally smoothly, without a hitch, and you can have your baby vaginally in a natural, superior way, most classes will reassure you. Unless you can't. The baby might turn, or stall. There might be fetal distress. For any number of reasons that might come up, there may be an intervention of some kind, whether to ease pain or correct a troubling issue, all the way up to a C-section. A good class is going to make you comfortable and knowledgeable about the many possibilities but ultimately reinforce that whatever happens, happens, and you need to be able to roll with that.

You Should Be in Sync with Your Care Provider

It's great that you and your partner, midwife, doula, mother-in-law, and best friend from kindergarten are all in this thing together. But what you really need to do is make sure you have a care provider who understands your ideal birth, is committed to working with you to make sure you get the healthiest version of that birth possible, and has fully explained to you what is possible and not possible.

> "Love is all fun and games until someone loses an eye or gets pregnant."
>
> —Jim Cole

Did you want to avoid an epidural at all costs, unless the pain becomes excruciating? Are you totally against an episiotomy? A good birthing class will get you thinking about these possibilities to open the door for conversations you should be having with your doctor before it's go time. And if you realize you aren't a good fit, you can change providers before it's too late. People do this! It seemed insane to me, but at least two women in my class realized their doctors' birthing techniques were far more C-section–oriented than they felt comfortable with, so they found more compatible providers.

A Birth Plan Is So Important, Except Not at All

You might want to write up a birthing plan that details what you mean by an ideal birth, which a birthing class should help you achieve by talking over what that could look like. It is good to visualize how you want it to go. But you also need to put your trust into the hands of your provider and let her drive the car, realizing that this is a glorified wish list and not a set-in-stone battle plan.

> **"I'm already pregnant, so what other kind of shenanigans could I get into?"**
>
> —Diablo Cody, *Juno: The Shooting Script*

A good birthing class will help you outline what you can really dig your heels in over when it comes to labor. For example, barring any medical issues, maybe you want to hold your baby immediately on your chest after you give birth, you want to try to nurse right away, or you want your baby in the recovery room with you at night. But you should also get a realistic sense of what you won't have much control over, which is damn near everything. If you're induced, you won't be moving around all that much. If you wanted a water birth, that can't happen when you're hooked up to an IV. These are important distinctions to know your way around to be your own best advocate.

Only Allow Helpful People in the Birthing Room

Just as your pregnancy is not the time to fraternize with bad vibes, the labor room is not the place for the judgy friend who loves you but always makes you feel kind of self-conscious; or the passive-aggressive mother-in-law; or the long-lost so-and-so who decided to show up now; or even your mother, who walks in with a look on her face like you're about to die.

It's up to you and you alone—not your husband, boyfriend, partner, sperm donor—who gets to be in that room with you. Your sister-in-law can be there if you say so, but not just because your husband says so. Your vagina = your guest list. A good birthing class will reinforce how critical this is, and how important it is for you to communicate to your nurses the names of the people who will be allowed to see you during this extremely private, vulnerable, only-these-two-people-can-touch-me time.

Pain Is Subjective

One woman's sigh is another woman's holy-shit-get-this-thing-out-of-me. What your body can handle is up to your body to decide. You can mind-over-matter it to a frighteningly awesome degree, but you are not David Blaine. Any good birthing class will stress a million times that your body is capable of far more than you realize—and it is, to a crazy, mind-blowing degree—but it will also not judge what a woman needs to get through labor, whether that's a doula, Dave Matthews Band, or an armful of Demerol.

Every Pregnancy Is Different

When you look around at the couples in your birthing class, you will quickly realize that everyone's pregnancy is different. Every couple's relationship is different. Everyone's birth plan is different. Some women are innately more comfortable in their pregnant bodies than others. Some women seem like naturals at this thing, while other women seem endlessly anxiety-ridden. There is no one way to feel about being pregnant, and a good birthing class will help you talk through all the fears and feelings a pregnancy can bring up. It will normalize those differences.

This is important to remember even if this isn't your first child. You may think you know exactly how your labor will go, but you will likely be totally wrong. Wrap your head around the fact that it probably won't be a rerun of your previous experience(s).

Coping Is Individual

If meditation isn't your thing, maybe focusing on breathing is. Maybe you love using that giant inflatable ball. A birthing class that's helpful will give you a grab bag of tools to manage the work of your labor, from breathing, to meditating, to position changing, to all sorts of coping mechanisms, so that you can pick what works for you in the moment.

> **"If pregnancy were a book they would cut the last two chapters."**
>
> —Nora Ephron, Julia Gilden's *Woman to Woman*

Things Aren't Always What They Seem

Birthing classes normalize differences, but they also highlight them. If you end up in a birthing class with a rock star and his lovely wife who seem like the perfect, happy expecting couple, you may learn by the class's end that the dude is kind of distant, the chick is still not eating enough, and they totally can't agree on exactly how natural the birth should be. Pregnancy is human vulnerability; it brings out crazy weird magnifications of your feelings and wishes and deepest notions, and it's fruitless to do anything but dive into your own pregnancy and not compare it to anyone else's. Your experience is yours.

Body Acceptance on Steroids

If you don't leave birthing class feeling like a light, floating cloud of totally validated human-ness who could go film a pregnancy-fetish porno immediately upon leaving class, you deserve your money back. Birthing classes are great for talking so freely and naturally about your body as an amazingly superior medical miracle that was made to do this, and it goes a long way toward loving your pregnant body. Your body is built to birth babies! You can handle whatever happens! You are a woman, and women give birth, and when it's time to get that baby out, out that baby will come! Out of you! Like a superwoman! You can do this! Naturally! Organically! And it is beautiful! Any birthing class that doesn't dole out exclamatory body acceptance in spades is doing it so wrong it is practically illegal.

There Is No Perfect Life in Which to Bring a Baby

Much as it might seem like it, that rock-star couple with the seemingly perfectly planned pregnancy, perfect minimal weight gain, and perfect white Volvo C30 were not planted in your birthing class for the express purpose of showing you what your life would look like if you had just "been more careful," waited one more year to get pregnant, saved more money, achieved more, and done this thing correctly, but that won't stop you from feeling that way.

If you could peel back the layers of their shiny existence, you'd see that she wants a hospital birth and he wants a home birth. He's always on the phone, and she is left to learn to hypnotize herself through the labor.

Whatever it really is, it's not your concern, and it's not your life for a reason. Be content in the knowledge that you will do this the only way you can. That's what a birthing class *should* teach you.

STAGE **4**:

EXCITEMENT

• • •

THE ACTUAL BABY ARRIVES!

22.

THE BABY IS COMING: A FEW THOUGHTS ON LABOR

If there was ever a time to lose the ambivalence about pregnancy and child-rearing and step up to the plate, go to bat, and an assortment of other relevant sports metaphors, it is now. Soon, you shall be called at a moment's notice to enter into battle for the birth of your baby. Trumpet blast: *Remember your training, soldier!*

Only, uh, you've really not had any specific training for this experience. Maybe you took a birthing class or twelve and have now been armed with tips out the wazoo. Maybe you've read ALL the books twice, and watched *Teen Mom, A Baby Story, Birth Day,* and *Bringing Home Baby* on repeat for months. Hell, maybe you owe TLC your future baby's first paycheck for all the help they've thrown your way learning about what goes down in the delivery room.

But this is all merely dress rehearsal for the real thing, and the thing about that real thing is that no class, book, or show can tell you what your specific labor will be like. This is not cause for alarm. It's cause for excitement! A real mystery! A real page-turner! In your actual life!

So take a moment and ponder these things during the very long, boring, anticipatory, exciting, frustrating, confusing, wonderful days and weeks before you go into battle, never to return as the same person again. Here are some key things to consider about this oh-so-precious time.

You Have Double the Blood Volume Right Now

This makes sense when you think about it, because you have a second person in there who needs her very own blood. But when you realize you are actually out there sloshing around pregnant with DOUBLE THE BLOOD VOLUME of a normal human, it's not exactly easy to stomach. My first response was, naturally: gag, gross, ick, eww. But then it just seemed fraught with danger, like one false move with a stapler and we'd have a gusher, a Slip 'N Slide of blood trailing behind me. I felt like a walking biohazard. It also felt really surreal, like a kind of tipping point of pregnant-ness.

You Are Maxed-Out Prego to the Max

You feel like a whale no matter how much weight you gained. The farts hit maximum torch peak. The heartburn is pure throat fire. You can't sleep. You have crazy dreams. You're so horny. You're so turned off. You feel like a croissant. But at least you literally can't be more pregnant than this, unless you're still pregnant for like another week or two.

Your Due Date Is a Guestimate

It almost rhymes. I know you know that your due date is a rough estimate of forty weeks from the time they think you conceived, but that won't stop you from freaking the fuck out when it rolls around and you are still a croissant with no baby to show for it. No matter how many times they tell you it's an estimate, or how many times you hear that it takes longer for first-time pregos to have their kid, you will treat that date like it's D-Day. It's not. In fact, since this pregnancy was unexpected, your dates might be even MORE of a guess than they would otherwise be.

Resist the urge to predict the time off you'll need, or walk out of your office after torching the place because you know you're not coming back. Also, unless you're on bed rest, you're probably still at work right now, which is probably the closest thing to hell you've ever experienced. If you're still working, believe me: it's the one thing helping you not go crazy because you haven't had this damn baby yet.

Everyone Is Annoying

Okay, maybe everyone was annoying the whole time you were pregnant, but now they are extra, special, totally, balls-out annoying. Do me a favor and write down every time someone says:

» "'Bout to pop, eh?"
» "When you gonna have that baby?"
» "Are you SURE there's only one in there?"
» "Haven't had that baby yet, huh?"
» "What will you do if your water breaks at work?"

Etc. People are so invested in how large (or not large) you are, and when you are going to have this baby. Not the caring for it or raising it or feeding it, per se, but the thing-coming-out-of-you part. It's just human. They can't help their gawking faces and slacking jaws. Try to pity them. Try to humor them. When all else fails, mock them outright. You're pregnant. Pregnant pass. Invoke it! Last chance!

You Will Get Super Puffy at the End

You are the Stay Puft Marshmallow Man at this point. You could roll around your house without even walking, so soft and puffy you are. It is a bizarre time in pregnancy when you look like you're permanently wearing a fat suit. Take a picture, hide that picture, and make sure you pull it out and laugh hysterically about it in three months.

Your Body Smells Weird

Showers get difficult at the end, what with the slippery tub, inability to see your lower extremities, and lack of adequate towel coverage. So why bother? Do bother. Do it for your loved ones and anyone within a 300-foot radius. Don't do what I did and have your entire pregnancy characterized by you smelling like chicken-noodle soup.

You Could Get Really Horny

Something about maxing out the absolute biological function of your body as a woman can feel really freeing. And if it doesn't, they say semen helps aid contractions, so do it for your baby. (Then again, they say that about spicy eggplant lasagna, too.)

You'll Wish It Was Winter

It's truly better to be massively pregnant in the winter, when the constant sweats will convince you that, if nothing else, pregnancy is some kind of foreshadowy prophecy of menopause. Only the really, really fertile kind.

You May Be Groped in Public at Any Time

Now that you're "about to pop," everyone you encounter will let you know. As if you didn't. But that doesn't hold a candle to how free complete strangers will feel to touch and probe you. Sometimes people want to FEEL YOUR BABY KICK. They mean well; allow the plebes to experience your miracle if you want to. Once, at a thrift store, a clerk reached over and started pressing just under and around my rib cage and let me know I was having a boy. (It was a girl.)

It Might Be Hard to Stop Eating

Even if you've been told to curtail the vacuuming of all nearby food-like items because you've gained too much weight, you might feel unable to do much about it. Why not have a snack? If you're going to have the baby any day now, what's one more bag of pepperonis? No, really, keep it light, keep it healthy, and keep yourself in the best state you can to get ready for the exertion of labor.

Walk. Just Walk.

Your best bet to get that baby out is to put the chicken leg down and walk. Walk like your life depended on it. Walk like you've been paid to do it. Walk like you're in a marathon to make babies come out. Walk like you're Forrest Gump, but walking.

(If It's Your First Baby) You'll Get So Bored

If this is your first baby, waiting around for her to decide when she feels like making her debut is about as exciting as a hernia. Meaning, it's literally painful and not fun. You'll get so bored that after you're done reorganizing your winter scarves into various placenta shapes, you'll start coming up with stupid ideas that seem super logical at the time. Like renting a cabin in the mountains the weekend your baby is due because you've decided that if you go out of town on a long road trip, that's like asking the baby to be born, so the baby will HAVE to start coming, because that would be so inconvenient as to work, RIGHT?!?! And then you'll do it, and on the second night, you'll start having crazy contractions, and you'll pack up and hop in the car and drive back home excitedly thinking that you did it, you really controlled this thing, those SUCKERS, and then the contractions . . . will stop. Yeah. Braxton Hicks, my friend.

The moral? Save your money. Wait it out. You can do this. Remember what I said about cashing in your free time? Do it until the last drop of your water has broken.

(If It's Not Your First Baby) You'll Want to Keep the Baby Inside as Long as Possible

If you have other children already, however, you know this: As difficult as pregnancy can be, babies are usually easier to take care of "on the inside." You can't hear them. They don't need to be actively fed. You don't need to use your arms to carry them. So enjoy the last days with your other children, who will immediately seem a) enormous and b) extremely self-sufficient when the baby arrives.

You Might Never Get the Nesting Instinct

Sure, you'll clean and organize and plan for your baby, but it's entirely possible you will never be struck down with the OCD need to scrub a kitchen floor or vacuum an attic. It's okay. But you'll definitely wish you had later when you and your baby arrive back at home and the first thing you notice is that disgusting kitchen floor.

It's the Most Exciting Unknown Ever

As tough as waiting on a baby can be, it's also ridiculously mysterious. What the hell is this thing going to look like? Be like? Feel like? Act like? How will your labor go? Will it be over fast? Will you break any records? Will you need painkillers? Will you rock it naturally?

You literally don't know any of this, much less when the baby will arrive. There's nothing you can do but second-guess contractions and eat spicy foods, except don't eat too much, and remember the thing about walking. It is agonizing, but then it really is over. And yet, you will always remember that anxiety and purgatory fondly.

In Goes One of You and Out Come Two

This is insane! Really sit with the idea that in no short order, this thing you've been growing, which becomes more real to you as every moment passes, is about to be outside of you. LIKE A PERSON. You're going to meet! You're going to get to know each other! Your life is changing irrevocably in a matter of days or hours. It is truly a diverging path.

23.

HOLY SHIT, YOU'RE IN LABOR

When you're actually in labor, you'll have another whole range of things to consider, such as . . .

Keep Your Mind as Open as Your Legs

There's no telling how your labor will go, and the best thing you can do is have a plan for that birth with a big, fat asterisk: whatever happens, you'll roll with it. It is the only way to not lose your mind when you find yourself needing that epidural you were never going to have, getting that C-section you didn't think would be necessary, etc. This is not the time for rigid adhesion to anything but the principle that having a healthy baby is the end goal. Save yourself a lot of agony and roll with it.

Even Though You're in Labor, There Could Be Long Periods of Complete Inactivity

You'll need that open mind when you discover that short of a few big moments, labor involves a lot of sitting, walking, lying, and otherwise waiting. Take comfort in the knowledge that it's the most boring exciting thing you'll ever do. In the meantime, don't be surprised if you labor through several nursing shifts, a three-day weekend, or spring.

Last Chance to Waste Time. Go!

But then again, this is the last time for a long time that you'll sit around doing nothing. Cherish it. Especially if you have other kids, since I'll assume someone else is watching them. Enjoy the "time off"!

Defend Your Turf

Remember, there are no bad vibes allowed in the room where you will meet your baby. Keep out anyone who isn't a pure heart or expression-free face, and never let them make you feel guilty for it.

You Will Poop. In Front of Everyone. It's Part of It.

Listen, honey, you're going to poop yourself while you're giving birth. Yes. You are. No. Nope. No, really, there's nothing you can do about it. Not even that. Yep. Uh-huh. YES. Duh, of course there will be people around. They're definitely going to see it. Someone has to wipe it. Yeah. It comes out of your butt right there in front of everyone. No, you can't really control how much. You won't even be able to tell. Yes, the nurses have seen it all before and could not care less. In fact, it helps them know that you're pushing correctly. And yeah, they won't tell you it's happening. You'll have to trust that your husband or boyfriend or girlfriend or friend will tell you if you did it. No, they'll never forget it either.

And the best part is that you won't even care.

Someone Will Smuggle You Some Food, and That Person Truly Loves You

Self-explanatory.

You might later hate that person if you barf up said food during labor, but in the moment, they have done a beautiful thing for you.

You're Not Done Yet!

After you're all done with pushing out your baby and you're super exhausted but happy and it's all surreal and wonderful, you won't actually be done with the whole thing yet. You still have to push out this other large beefsteak-type thing called the placenta. It usually only takes a few minutes after the baby is born before it comes out, and rest assured that it should not be as painful as your baby-pushing contractions. In comparison, these mild placenta cramps will feel like a gentle spring breeze blowing through your vagina.

Also, they might show the placenta to you. I remember distinctly that mine looked like a hot water bag, but made of organ.

Weight-Loss Confusion

You'll be shocked and surprised when you give birth, but you'll still somehow look like you're in your second trimester. It's fluid. It's swelling. It's gas. Basically, it's still a hot mess in there, even though the baby has vacated the premises.

Rest assured, things will return to some semblance of normal relatively soon. In the meantime, don't burn your maternity leggings just yet.

Hormone Crash = Circus Act

Fresh off the high of post-delivery euphoria, the last thing you will be thinking about from your intensive "what happens when I'm in labor" reading or classes is that this slaphappy buzz will soon do a nosedive. Yep, you are Wall Street, 1928, lady. And if it hits you really hard like it did me, you might immediately go reread those chapters in your little pregnancy book library, to try to make sense of this crazy fluctuation, and discover that they may not have painted an accurate portrait.

You might feel a little different or a little low, the books said, but then everything evens out, you have a soda, and the sun shines. But the reality is that you might totally find yourself through the roof with happiness one day and then paralyzed in the shower the next because you are sobbing uncontrollably for no reason. And this could go on for a miserable number of weeks. It would be one thing if everyone around you was like "Oh, right, the hormones! This is normal; don't worry! You're okay!" But this level of intuition and comfort cannot always be expected from the clerk at the local CVS.

Swiffer Pad

Obviously it makes sense you'll be bleeding after giving birth—how could you not? Not obvious at all is that the pad they will hand you to soak it up comes in one size, one industrial-strength, giant-pizza size, which is larger than any diaper you've ever imagined. I saved one of these pads for posterity. It is seriously bigger than a Swiffer pad. And I wanted to keep my commemorative Swiffer pad throughout several moves so whenever my girlfriends came over and talked about their future possible pregnancies I could whip it out, set it down quietly on the coffee table, and walk away. Nearly three years later, this has still not come up, but I always have it at the ready.

Burning Pee and Other Fun Postpartum Side Effects

To this day I feel completely uncomfortable with how much it burned when I peed after birth, and how nothing at all seemed to make it feel any better, and how nothing I read ever even seemed to mention this horrific side effect, and how it lasted for like two weeks. Painkillers might have helped, only my decision to go au naturel meant I had hippie midwives who were stingy with the stuff. I understand why, in retrospect—you don't need a nursing mother addicted to painkillers. But, oh, how I longed for anything to dull that weeks-long sizzle.

The beautiful part about childbirth is that every woman goes in with her own unique set of expectations, and every woman leaves with her own story, not to mention her own list of shocking aftereffects she feels unprepared for. I'd love to chalk it up to the pregnancy industrial complex, like some kind of conspiracy theory to keep women in the dark. But in reality it's that pregnancy really is so individual, and that there's no telling how your body will respond to the challenge. Think of your list of horrors as a kind of battle scar. And make sure that you do everyone a favor and share it every chance you get. Give to the quilt of pregnancy horror stories until it's big enough to warm us all.

It Is Still, Hands Down, the Most Awe-Inspiring Thing You'll Ever Do

I know, it's weird. How can anything so uncomfortable, so terrifying, so boring, so gross, be so beautiful and precious and gag-inducingly perfect? Nature wins. It's a high unmatchable by any drug, a happiness impossible to recreate through any other means, a truly path-diverging moment in your life. You are going in a pregnant lady and coming out a mother, and you will never ever be able to think of your self apart from that identity again. Yes, you'll still be you, and you'll still do other things and achieve wholly individual goals apart from childrearing, and some of them will even be fun. But that baby has your heart for good.

24.

WELCOME TO YOUR NEW, CLICHÉ-RIDDEN LIFE

Imagine if someone invited you to hang out for a weekend with the following activity menu:

Friday: Lift squirming watermelons
Saturday: Sob hysterically in shower
Sunday: Lunge ravenously at tossed slices of pizza

If it weren't for the pizza, I seriously doubt you'd agree. And yet, this is a typical weekend in the life of a mother with a newborn, assuming you can even make time for a shower. It's true: All that stuff about poop, drool, and lack of sleep is now yours to behold! Welcome to the club! Make it count! Put a rainbow on it! You did it!

It won't be easy, of course, given how many exclamation points I just used, but also because of how soul-numbing those first few weeks and months of no sleep and frequently ordered pizza can be. Not to mention that, unlike in college, this time you'll realize that pizza really does get old, even the wood-fired, artisan kind from the new hipster Italian place that knows how to make it *bianche.*

Whenever I see fresh new mothers with their fresh new babies, the mothers are actually never all that fresh and new. So I look for signs of the old person in there, the one who used to at least read magazines? Perhaps she's trapped, I think, screaming on the inside, dying to get out. She'll give me a nod or a wink as a signal, or perhaps pass me a slip of paper asking for help on my way to the bathroom? Never happens. She's stuck in this early-motherhood realization that it's not all rainbows and sunshine, and I can't help her out of it.

The work of caring for other people is difficult and thankless; otherwise it would be everyone's idea of a great job. Instead, it's almost no one's idea of exciting. So I had to roll my eyes when I saw all the pictures of other people's newborns on my Facebook feed, with parents beaming with love and pride, posting every single update on the journey of human growth along the way as if it's a privilege to change a diaper or clean spitup, with nary a mention that this stuff is, you know, hard?

I was fascinated by my baby, totally in love, totally curious about what she was doing and the motivation behind her every utterance. But I expected at least someone out there in Facebook land to give it up and mention the lack of sleep, for the love of God, the lack of sleep. But all I saw was the hashtag #perfect with every scroll.

If it feels like this is designed to make you feel like a horrible person with a heart two sizes too small who can't hang with the mundane stuff, congratulations; you are totally almost human.

The baby part is really precious, though. Here are the clichés that never feel clichéd, because they really are marvels of human aliveness. Watching her do stuff. Move around. Open her eyes. Look at me. Learning to nurse. Learning to be alive. It's crazy! Miracle of life, you guys! That shit is real! But, of course, the shit is also real. Your heart will do a lot of melting and swelling and thumping, all for this tiny little creature whose gifts come in many forms, including tiny little deposits in her diaper.

"If your baby is beautiful and perfect, never cries or fusses, sleeps on schedule and burps on demand, an angel all the time, you're the grandma."

—Theresa Bloomingdale

The rest of it is about as exciting as watching your taxes being filed (minus the crushing fear that you're about to have to cough up a grand or four). Maybe those of us who feel this way are defective mutants who don't know how to love (we do; it's just not like in commercials).

Maybe our lack of planning just means we didn't have a chance to build up the experience so much in our minds, so that when it became reality, we were missing that rehearsed gratitude and magic and wonder to buffer it. Who can learn to "live in the moment" on the spot when the moment is comprised of incessant crying?

That said, it's not really all that bad. Really. Somehow, you kinda get used to the little bugger. Your brain figures out how to stop distinguishing the precious baby from her care, to settle into the combination of beautiful and exhausting they present together. They are, in fact, inextricable, and it is in the caring that you're doing most of the loving. Weird.

And along the way, you'll pick up a trick or two to get yourself through this massive, unending series of clichés called Raising an Infant, part technique and part attitude adjustment. It's totally okay if you never learn to like this part. But even if you don't, you may find out that somewhere in there inside you is a person who just changed ten diapers in one day and did not even sorta feel like dunking your head into the diaper pail.

A few tips . . .

Caffeine and Ibuprofen

Don't go crazy on the stuff, especially if you're nursing, because that's just undoing the whole point of taking this stuff in the first place by keeping your baby up and jittery, giving you more work to do. But in order to go into this thing armed with anything like a buffer from how raw these first few weeks and months can feel, I suggest getting real acquainted with the perks of caffeine and ibuprofen. They'll smooth out those edges, keep those trains moving, and overall slap a coat of oil on those rusty joints. Once you've got that down, it will be so much easier to face the trials and tribulations with good, old-fashioned grit and moxie.

Diaper Delight

The one saving grace to changing so many freaking diapers in those early weeks and months is that you can focus instead on the fact that your baby's poop is like a little thermometer of her health. Marvel at this impromptu lesson in human soiling. You don't have to obsess over it—some people actually do that! Please don't do that!—but you should be cognizant that pee and poop are happening for a reason, because they're directly tied to hydration and eating.

The second you roll up to your pediatrician or dial the on-call nurse hotline, they are going to ask about this activity. So it's important to pay attention. No, I would not go so far as to suggest that the monitoring of diapers is fun or anything, but I promise you that you have not correctly anticipated how fascinating it actually is. I figure if you realize that what's in them isn't useless either, you might fight through the (literal) funk in the name of good parenting.

If you get really bored by it anyway, and you want a REAL challenge, give yourself the mind-melting task of trying to determine which saves more in money, energy, and effort: cloth or plastic. It seems so easy to figure out! It's just a simple calculation! Said all the newborn mothers found rocking in the corner with a calculator and a copy of their latest water bill.

Nursing/Feeding

These are two entirely different experiences, of course, but both tend to be just as frequent, not to mention challenging, especially when you're doing it around that clock, to the tune of ten to 287 times a day.

Whether you are struggling to get the latch right for breastfeeding or sterilizing bottle nipples until your eyes bleed, it's important to remind yourself that what you're doing here is helping to make that poop you'll be so excited to see/smell later. This is the front end of the factory! This is the keeping-the-baby-alive part! This stuff is a lab experiment in efficiency and human bonding! Viewed from that angle—whichever angle involves sitting down—it's hard to get too grumpy about it.

This is also a rare chance for one of those postcard moments you see so often in cultural depictions of motherhood: a moment of utter serenity, peace, quiet. It really can be like that. Not always, of course. Sometimes you'll instead experience the deeply rewarding pleasure of a fussy baby spitting white goo into your hair while you sob hopelessly. Or, you know, if you're struggling to get your baby to take the damn bottle, then it is and can be a frustrating game of How Else Can I Do This Wrong? you'll be playing ten times a day. Oh, the moments.

But once you get the hang of these moments, man, you are one badass-feeling motherfucker. You just got the holy grail of motherhood down. You are Indiana Jones, and you just reclaimed your hat. You are Kathleen Turner holding the jewel of the Nile, by God. You are Lara Croft, and this is an ancient artifact up in this piece! This is *The Hunger Games*, and you are—no, too violent. Anyway, you have nourished your child! The goal of the ancients! Revel in the feeling of having successfully done what all humans since the dawn of time are, in a sense, meant to do: usher in the next generation.

Lack of Sleep

Granted, the first night it's kinda fun. Exciting, even. Like a slumber party. You've arrived home from the hospital and here is your newborn child, and of course you're ready to welcome her home and get to know each other. You roll through night one like a champ. *I got this one!* you exclaim proudly.

Unfortunately, it's never exciting again, not even once, not even for a second. By night two, you're kind of a grouch. By night three, you're an all-out dick about it. And by night four, you and whoever is winging this thing with you are complete lunatics, stumbling around out there trying to buy the correct kind of bottle inserts, and things get mixed up and people snap at each other and before you know it you are sleep-hissing. Yes, sleep-hissing.

Sleep-hissing is a serious problem for couples with newborns, who, out of their minds with lack of sleep and no relief, must resort to communicating by hissing at each other while their baby sleeps tenuously in the next room (or same room, or same bed) so as not to wake her. Do you know what sleep-hissing sounds like? Like two people who hate each other so much they would rather not even speak at audible volumes. It is all barely contained rage with none of the positive attributes of actual human speech. Make no mistake: You don't actually hate anyone. But that is what lack of sleep is going to do to you.

The only way I could get through this unbelievably cruel stupor was to pretend I was being tortured and had to stay alive. I pretended I was trapped in a game called You Will Never Sleep Again. Much like getting used to round-the-clock feedings, I had to pretend I was some kind of captured assassin or top-secret operative in training who had to tough this out to prove that I was worthy of this role. I was Jason Bourne, and these motherfuckers—whoever they were didn't really matter, but if you need a solid visual, I suggest picturing Alan Rickman—would not get the best of me.

Strangely, it totally worked, and as I imagined I would get no sleep, every hour or two here or there was not a reason for grouchiness but a godsend. A charge-up to get me through the next few hours. Give it a try. Of course, if that fails, try pretending that you are in a play about someone who is chronically hung over and has to raise a child. That is also eerily easy to do.

In truth, I've still probably not completely recovered from my own time in the sleepless, nonstop feeding and diaper-changing trenches. Lack of sleep is no joke. It does not fuck around. You will try to search your brain for a time when you remembered being this tired, like when you would pull an all-nighter or suffer from a bout of insomnia. The thing is, though, you can take medication to get through insomnia, and the all-nighter you usually chose to do all on your own! Knowing you would have something called a "weekend" during which you might "catch up" on sleep.

There is no such thing in your life anymore. You are experiencing "forced sleeplessness"—suffering because another human being, your baby, has decided that if she's up, everybody is up! And she will decide that approximately every forty-six minutes. Or less.

The Perilous Flash-Forwards

It's probably for good reason—like to frighten you into being hypervigilant about choking hazards—but that doesn't make it any less terrifying when your brain starts doing *Terminator*-style paranoia scans of every room and situation you are in to imagine the worst-case scenario for you.

What this could mean is that when you, say, carry your baby outside, your brain might flash a scene of you dropping her and watching her head bust open on the asphalt driveway. Or when you open the freezer while holding your baby, you imagine what would happen if you just happened to trip, chucking her up and into the freezer, where, for some inexplicable reason, she becomes trapped inside.

It is morbid as all get-out, and yet, apparently, it's totally normal. And the injury doesn't even seem to have to be a logical or even likely possibility. But that doesn't stop your brain from showing you the most horrifying, tragic possibilities in every uncovered electrical socket, every sharp corner, every unsecured bookcase.

For weeks, I struggled with these flash-forwards. Was it postpartum depression? Some kind of psychosis? I wasn't hearing voices, or being instructed to DO these things to my baby. I loved my baby. I just couldn't stop imagining her death from injury, as if suddenly I'd brought her home to a haunted house of carnival terrors.

Eventually, I started to see them as merely information with really good special effects. In a way, it was kind of great to feel like a vigilant seer of baby hazards, even if it meant I had to shudder at the thought of what the reality of such an injury could look like. Then, I finally asked my husband if the same thing was happening to him. I guess I'd waited so long because I didn't want to admit I was imagining horrible things. But I was relieved when he confessed he had been getting the same flash-forwards. We were able to laugh about how terrifying it is to walk around with the equivalent of your own version of *Final Destination* starring your baby playing in your head 24-7.

Luckily, our baby never did experience anything like a serious injury in the first year of her life, but between the perilous flash-forwards and the SIDS risk, we were more than happy to take things a bit cautiously.

. . .

What seemed like a very long time ago, you were just you. An autonomous person moving around with a body you could call your own. Now you have multiplied. And there is literally a baby outside of your body that you can call your own. No, seriously, whether you like it or not, it's now yours, like a handbag, except the handbag is a living, breathing thing.

Funny enough, in a few years you'll be far out of those woods and into new ones. But when you look back at this tenuous time, they will seem mercifully foggy. You will hardly remember the aching pain, the torturous exhaustion. You'll just remember the fog, the distant hazy fog, and the zombie-like way you moved through your life, somehow managing to make appointments, keep a job, and operate heavy machinery. This, too, is for a reason. So that when some random lady with a baby on the way asks you what it's like in the beginning, while you juggle a purse, child, diaper bag, and a *bianche*, you'll answer without skipping a beat and actually mean it: it's not that bad.

25.

GET USED TO FEELING LIKE SHIT FOR A WHILE

Tender is the night now that you just had a baby, and so is your vagina. You are settling into the routine of your little one's care. But what about you? And more importantly, what happened to your body? Your body is a wonderland, all right, but it's not the John Mayer–infused kind.

I don't know why no one just comes right out and says it: You're going to feel like shit after you have your baby. Is it because they don't feel like shit? It can't be true. Your back hurts, your hips hurt, your legs hurt, your vagina hurts, your vulva hurts, your tits hurt, your feet hurt, your head hurts, your arms hurt, everything you can think of hurts, and it also hurts to think.

You don't poop right, fart right, pee right, or bleed right. Your hair falls out; you piss yourself; your back fuckin' kills. All you want is to get back to normal poop-pee-hair-back as fast as possible, but what the hell is normal anyway, and can you ever really go home again? The answer is no. But you can sure as hell try.

"Remember this, for it is as true as true gets: Your body is not a lemon. You are not a machine. The Creator is not a careless mechanic. Human female bodies have the same potential to give birth well as aardvarks, lions, rhinoceri, elephants, moose, and water buffalo. Even if it has not been your habit throughout your life so far, I recommend that you learn to think positively about your body."

—Ina May Gaskin, *Ina May's Guide to Childbirth*

Sure, since we didn't plan our pregnancies, we were sucker-punched by more than just heartburn—we missed the chance to get ahead of the game on having a low-impact pregnancy, at least when it comes to exercise and weight gain.

If you avoided gaining a lot of weight, it will be easier to lose the weight, if for no other reason than there won't be as much to lose. If you exercised before you got pregnant and during the pregnancy, it will be easier to start exercising, as opposed to doing it, say, for the first time since high school, now that you're thirty-four. But if you weren't on top of those things because this pregnancy came out of left field, it's that much harder to deal with them postpartum.

But you'll be pleased to find out that most women are equally screwed postpartum in nearly every other way. Whether you had a C-section or a vaginal birth, the recovery time—six weeks or so—is roughly the same, and the differences between how long it takes to fart right again are individual. What, if anything, can you do about it then?

Be Good to Yourself

It's important to treat yourself well after you give birth. Pretend you are Cleopatra, or the Queen of Sheba, or one of those women in the old Calgon commercials. Envision whomever you need to let yourself rest as much as possible. Yes, this is nearly impossible. But five minutes of a good foot rub or a four-minute shower or new PJs against your tired, old-lady body does wonders. Buy the good green tea. Eat the expensive cinnamon chocolate. Do little things whenever you can to make yourself feel better. It is so, so helpful in those early weeks and doesn't even have to cost a lot.

Never Refuse Help

When you feel like shit and you look like it, too, it's probably easier and very tempting to tell everyone you are fine and can handle it, so don't stop by. But one hour of someone playing with your kid while you take a bath is magic. Never underestimate what a quick drive to town to get your favorite coffee while someone walks your baby can do for a quick energy boost. Just make sure when someone offers to help, she is really going to help and not just come over and talk about work gossip while you struggle to nurse. That is just stressful. Instead, choose a specific task that person can do.

Go Easy on Yourself

Okay, so your body doesn't look like it did on prom night, and it didn't look like that on prom night either. You'll live, and it will change. If you have to ignore your body for a few weeks, do that. If you have to think of it as a utilitarian workhorse, do that. If you have to think of it as a rectangle made of wet cat food, so be it. Put it out of your mind; put it on another plane. Focus on the now, and think about your body when you have the time and energy to do something about it.

Walk. Go Outside. Move.

You're not Gwyneth Paltrow (right?!) or Kate Hudson, so you don't have to get your pre-pregnant body back in under thirteen hours. You have time. Start small, at whatever level matches your energy. If that means going for walks around the block with the baby, limit yourself to that. If you can run, pick up the pace. Do whatever kind of movement feels good. Just do something. It will build back to a more comfortable pace, and you'll feel less like a cat-food blob every day. Plus, you need the vitamin D, and if your baby is breastfed, so does he/she.

Have a Sense of Humor about It

If those hamhocks need to lie out in the sun for a few minutes, by all means, get them roasting. If your boobs feel like two soggy cantaloupes, say so. What is missing in the body-acceptance conversations in lady circles is the idea that you can laugh at your imperfections, and it's perfectly healthy. Sure, it can go too far if it prevents you from really liking what you see, or if it's just a defense mechanism to hide insecurity. But I think laughing about the sack of rusty mufflers you now call your body will help you take it all with a large block of salt. Just don't be too funny because it probably hurts your vulva to laugh. Plus, you're going to piss yourself. And that's gonna burn.

Take Your Time Getting Back on the Horse

I don't care what anyone else does. Reconnect with yourself at your pace, in your own way, and on your own schedule. This is not a race to look like the old you; it's a transformation to a different, new person who is probably terrifying at first but, in the end, might feel like a much better fit. Since this pregnancy was unexpected, this transformation might take longer than you think. That's okay. Don't rush it.

But When You Do Get Back on the Horse, Go All In

When you do start to feel more like your old self again, seize the day. You have no idea how long a good sleeping routine will last, how long until the next teething phase strikes. This means if you see a window for getting fit, taking a yoga class, focusing on your nutrition, then immerse yourself like it's time to learn traveler's Italian. You have no idea when your next window will open.

Take in Every Moment with Your Baby

Speaking of open windows, in spite of how utterly weird it is to be so broken-feeling physically but so desperately needed at the same time, loving that baby is a great antidote to the physical discomfort healing brings. What is pretty impressive is how much you will master transcending the sleeplessness, the hunger, the weird contortion of the only nursing position that your baby seems to like, and the clinginess.

And when you do that, you are in a bubble of baby time. You are looking at a tiny creature that you made, and you can marvel, learn, and love him/her. And you will see that even as caring for a newborn can deplete you, it is like a protein bar for your bruised, battered body.

26.

MANAGING VISITORS THE FIRST FEW WEEKS HOME

In the midst of those foggy early days of newborn care, you may find yourself worrying over a different guest list altogether: who to let hang out with you and your newborn those first few weeks.

This shit matters. These are the first days your baby spends in her new home. These are the first nights you and yours sleep with your child where you live, in the place she may very well grow up. It's about new rituals, new meetings, new experiences, and you want it to be sweet and poignant and lovely.

Sure, that poignant loveliness might come laced with a super grouchy irritability. You're dealing with hormone crashes, actual physical pain, weird things coming out of weird places, completely displaced internal organs, and a butt that hurts to sit on. You're learning an entirely foreign concept on the fly, trial by fire, and no amount of books can predict your baby's habits exactly, or what it takes to calm her.

You need some basic help, and you need it from someone who understands you are in many ways still in labor: You want someone to give you everything you need while not actually touching you. So while you're changing out that Swiffer pad, dagger-peeing, nursing, and trying to get a routine down, you'll be managing your kickball team of visitors for those first few critical days and weeks, and usually that means close relatives and friends, coworkers, etc. They all want to "help," and you should be grateful, but anyone who says "help is help" has never been helped wrong.

There are a few things to consider:

The Learning Curve

While you're lying in the hospital aching like someone who just fell off a bike directly onto her vagina, you won't realize how spoiled you've already gotten. There are nurses on call at the touch of a button, around the clock, to help you feed, bathe, and rock your baby to sleep. If you're nursing, someone can actually watch the baby sleep and then bring him to you to feed. Imagine the possibilities! In real life, this is called a night nurse, and I have heard it is a wonderful thing.

Once you're back at home, the hospital honeymoon is over, and you can certainly push buttons all day long, but no one will come, or they will just be your husband's emotional ones. It's time to figure out this baby on your own turf.

In this situation, whomever you choose to help during this time should be someone who will teach you a thing or two about babies. If this is your first baby, your learning curve will be steep, so you need someone to help you along. My mother-in-law had raised two children in the 1980s, which means she still understood what diapers looked like and knew how to hold a baby's head. These things are key.

Anyone who is going to argue with you about how to diaper or clean a baby until you're in tears and hate yourself should only be a benchwarmer unless there's a real serious drought of first-stringers.

Nursing

If you breastfeed, this is the first time you have to really get nursing going on your own, all by yourself, just you and your baby staring each other down, vying for dominance. If you were still working this out while in the hospital, and there's a good chance you will go home still working it out, this can be a very vulnerable, frustrating time.

The last thing you need around is someone who thinks boobs are funny or gross, or that nursing is weird. Worst of all is someone who is super inhibited, because the boobs are going to be coming out and they are going to be staying out. You'll cover them up for certain company, but the having out of the boobs is a key thing to rocking nursing, so pick someone who isn't squeamish about cantaloupes.

Chef Surprise

If you have a mother or mother-in-law visiting to help, it's likely she will cook for you. This is a godsend. Being well and warmly fed during those first few weeks without having to lift a finger to the dish soap goes a long way toward supplying the comfort and nourishment you need to get back on your feet.

It's pretty much win-win unless she makes all your most-loathed dishes. Whoever is related to the cook must advise of dietary or preference concerns in advance. Also, a note about your diet and nursing: Make sure the cook is going to load you up with extra servings for those 500 calories more you'll need to get a milk supply going. But if they start to load you up with milk-inhibiting foods that will make your baby a gassy jerk for her first week of life—garlic broccoli surprise— you have my permission to sob, sulk, or protest, whichever takes less energy.

Old Ways vs. New

An experienced mom can be a boon to a new mother who has only seen newborn babies on television. Experienced mothers are a sure hand when it comes to rocking a baby to sleep, or diagnosing colic. But make sure that helper is up to date. If she insists that all it takes to get your baby to sleep is a spoonful of whiskey, a shot of codeine, and an electric blanket, rethink your strategy.

Social Planner

It's great to have a helper to field visitors and requests to see you and the baby while you get used to this new life. Make sure it's someone who understands that those early visits should be short and sweet, and on the new parent's schedule. Nothing like parading your baby around to an endless stream of strangers and hangers-on who bring along the latest flu virus to you and the newbie.

Privacy

While "hanging out on your couch, nodding off, to deal with the fresh hell of sleeplessness" describes most of your days post-baby, on occasion you'll need to slip away for a bath or a nap or a moment of alone time. Choose a grown-up, autonomous guest who will respect your privacy and can hang out with your baby or on his own while reading and watching television. This seems like a no-brainer until you realize that hosting friends and coworkers who might have no idea how to act with a baby either is actually more exhausting than having the baby, because now you're busy entertaining two people, and one of them is hungry and didn't even bring you a casserole.

Proper Visit Length

Plan the length of time your visitors will stay ahead of time, so that you can adjust to the help without suffering from TLTE syndrome, short for They Left Too Early. You'll realize this the first time you need to take a shower and your husband is back at work and you realize you didn't actually devise a strategy to monitor the baby while also showering. On the other hand, you don't want your mother to still be sleeping on the couch when the baby starts kindergarten. It's hard to know in advance, but try to find a happy medium where you get the help you need but can also start your life on your own before too long.

. . .

The good news is that even if you have no help at all, you will figure things out. You will bring the baby seat into the bathroom and keep the curtain partially open. You will learn how to nurse a baby while mowing the lawn. You will discover that you can actually read a book out loud and pay attention to the History Channel. But until then, any and all shortcuts you can get are invaluable. Even if they are invaluable in teaching you what *not* to do.

27.

WHAT TO WEAR POSTPARTUM

While you were pregnant, you could conveniently use the fact that you were growing a person to justify the denim overalls, the sparkly moon boots, the ill-chosen floral smock. Now that you've had your baby, you have no such excuse, says everyone in your head. How do you return to the world in clothes that fit, look good, hide what ails you, and celebrate what's new in the middle of a newly mommed fashion purgatory? Maternity clothes? Old wardrobe? Hazmat suit? Welcome to your latest fashion dilemma, that tenuous time when you're semi-obviously no longer pregnant but it remains to be seen if you can snap back to the old you, the one who wore midriffs and tunics, or at least could have worn them if you'd felt like, by God.

And whereas you had nine long-ish months to accumulate that extra toddler or two in weight gain, you're now in a sudden race against time to relocate your old body, or at least that's how it feels. Where exactly did you leave that thing again? It might as well be in that box in your closet right next to your prom dress, since the chances of getting back into it are about as good as you slipping into a prairie-style Gunne Sax number by Jessica McClintock.

And of course, all this pressure to look nonpregnant comes at the time in your life when your body happens to feel . . . blobby. What you really don't need is pressure, self-inflicted or otherwise, to reappear through a cloud of smoke looking magically as you did that weekend you got knocked up. Instead, you need a guide to what to actually wear during all the phases just after birth, when your body is a Claymation surprise and your favorite new accessory is your baby, who happens to function as a kind of built-in art project for everything you put on. Better to map out some kind of strategy, because otherwise, it's your farted-up maternity pants every day for the whole next year. (Although some of us call the latter a win-win.)

The First Weeks Home

You've just returned home and it's time to start the recovery process while also diving head-first into a completely new, constantly disrupted schedule. It's not a time for vanity.

General Rule: Wear only what would feel really good to sleep or paint in and you're golden.

What That Looks Like: Go super easy on yourself in roomy yoga pants, sweats, carpenter pants, soft skirts, or even a maternity maxi dress. You'll also need something that won't impede changing a lot of pads or peeing with ease, and bonus points if it contains enough extra fabric to fan your bum with, on account of how much it burns when you pee after birth, which could be from stitches or a stretched-out vulva.

Keep everything boob-friendly upstairs with nursing tanks or T-shirts, because whether you go breast or bottle, your boobs need the space to breathe and swell. And throb, and ache, and deflate . . . If you're nursing, you need to be able to get those boobs out and fast, so just go ahead and make everything loose, comfy, and designed for maximum access. Nursing bras are worth every penny. If you're bottle-feeding, give yourself time to get back to a more stable size before dropping mad dough on expensive bras. In the meantime, go soft sports bra or go cheap.

Wiggle Room: This period in your life can be characterized by wearing literally the same outfit every single day for a few weeks (*cough* yoga pants and tank tops *cough*), and anyone who tries to tell you otherwise can go straight to hell right through the Forever 21 dumpster they crawled out of.

The First Trips Out

Eventually, you'll have to leave the house for something: diapers, groceries, a visit with a friend who insists on seeing your baby but for some insane reason can't come to your house, or, God forbid, returning to work. Time to step up the attire one tiny notch.

General Rule: Casual but slightly considered.

What That Looks Like: Even though you can drop several pounds in the hospital, what with the placenta, the baby, the water weight, the sweating, and the fact that they won't let you eat while you labor, you are still very likely to find a good, solid friend in those maternity pants you've been wearing this whole time. Aren't you glad you dropped some money on the good ones? Because with a new-and-improved, deflated midsection, these things still pass for jeans you could actually leave the house in, and who wants to run out and buy new jeans when you have no idea how quickly you're going to lose this weight? Baby ain't the only person who could use a security blanket.

Go for the maternity jeans and loose-fitting, comfortable, but flattering tops that make you feel like the best version of yourself you can be with a burning vulva. Hopefully this is just going to cover you for a few minutes at the post office, a trip to the grocery store, or a run-in at the coffee shop. Regardless, you need to be prepared to bump into your partner's ex, you know, the Medusa who said you were just a baby-hungry spinster who got knocked up on purpose? Making a tiny amount of effort for the first time after the baby comes actually makes you feel good and reminds you that sooner than you realize, you'll be back on your feet like old times. Ish.

Wiggle Room: If your baby is going with you on this trip, don't bother even changing your shirt covered in spit-up, because a newborn is basically like a portable poster board that announces, "Don't Have to Give a Shit About the Shirt." However, if you are out on your own, there's nothing whatsoever to indicate that at home is a writhing, wiggling little house of fluids, and who wants to keep repeating loudly to complete strangers that you just had a baby?

As the Weight (Finally) Falls

Joyous are the days you discover that the weight is actually coming off, without you doing anything but not sleeping and trying to determine whether your new baby's mystifying cries meet the medical definition of colic or if she just has really bad gas. Maddening are the long stretches of complete, utter, mystifying stasis, when you realize you'll actually have to move around to drop these pounds. If you're breastfeeding, keep in mind this hilarious tidbit: Lots of women can't keep the weight on while they breastfeed, while some of us are holding onto those pounds like they were personal love letters signed by *Chocolat*-era Johnny Depp. Either way, it's likely to be a weird time weight-wise, where you don't know what to expect from one week to the next.

General Rule: Whatever it takes to get you out of maternity clothes and into the new you, without dropping a bunch of dough on something you'll wear for only six weeks, is going to be one step toward feeling like less of a general blobby and more of a woman-shaped blobby that you used to know.

What That Looks Like: There's no telling how this will go. If you have the time to work out for six hours a day for six months straight like Kate Hudson, sure, don't even bother buying a transitional wardrobe; just march right up to your personal shopper and make her order a custom-made wardrobe to fit for the next two hours. If you work out some but not that regularly, because HELLO you just had a baby, things may not snap back like they do in Barbieland.

If the weight feels stubborn—and believe me, you'll know it—you do have some options if you want to ditch the maternity wear. Let's be honest, though: Those elastic-waistband mama pants were the best you ever had. It will be hard to let go. Regular jeans and pants with metal buttons will not only feel restrictive but sometimes even practically violent, and you'll find yourself dreaming of that time in the not-so-distant past when you could just slide up that band and keep on breathin'. You might even start to wonder if just getting pregnant again immediately would be worth it if only it meant you could put off regular pants for another two to three years.

You can absolutely keep rocking maternity clothes as long as you need to, but with one caveat: a muumuu is a muumuu is a muumuu. And while some maternity gear totally passes as business-casual, most of it screams loose-fitting polyester mom-core. It can become a kind of self-defeating state-of-mind thing, where as long as you're wearing maternity skirts with a waistband the size of a pillowcase, you're still a foreigner in your own country.

If this malaise sets in, consider a transitional wardrobe. It will set you back a few bones, but if it's the one-time purchase-bridge that transports you back to your old clothes in no time, it's probably worth it. For some of us, that wardrobe can look like a series of Russian nesting dolls that slowly shrink down to our old size over the course of months or years.

For me, this period looked something like this: I marched into Urban Outfitters and bought the skinny black cigarette pants in the almost-largest size they had. They were $50. I wore these until they were loose in a weird way, and then I went back and bought the next smaller size. And so on. Three sizes down, I am now one size bigger than where I was before I was pregnant. My baby turns three in a few months. Not three months. Three years.

I also kept wearing maternity tops throughout breastfeeding, which lasted well past the year I'd expected and all the way up to two and a half years. In between, I bought a few really cheap T-shirts and sweaters to fill in the gaps, but otherwise I deserve some kind of award for stubborn devotion to not buying any new clothes for almost three years.

Wiggle Room: Because this is an anything-goes kind of time, by all means, do whatever it takes to make you feel good. Post-pregnancy weight loss is so individual, so maddening, so simple, so complicated, especially when you throw nursing into the equation, that it's best to stick with whatever makes the most financial, comfort-level, and feel-good sense for you and tell everyone who has a problem with it to stick it up their Bella Band.

When You Want to Feel Good

In spite of how you feel at this particularly moment, you might actually want to take your rusty-muffler body out on the town for a spin. How best to sand-and-seal that puppy so it will gleam in the city lights?

General Rule: Black is best, stretchy fabrics are forgiving, and the rest is magic none of us can explain.

What That Looks Like: Maxi dresses are worth their maternity weight in gold, because many of them look like a floaty, beachy dream someone like Sade would wear. And they can be worn with the confidence of anyone who doesn't feel like they've pulled a magic trick worthy of David Blaine. There are some great stretchy maternity tops that accentuate the extremely generous cleavage you are probably displaying right now, and that can be paired with any number of cute maternity or regular jeans, or flowy skirts.

Wiggle Room: Don't do anything that's going to hurt your vulva. No night is worth that. In fact, "don't hurt your vulva" is really the only rule that matters in any of this.

28.

BREASTFEEDING: KIND OF A BITCH

Part of the excitement and awe of giving birth is the built-in knowledge that the pain and suffering will soon be over. That is, until you begin the often excruciatingly difficult process of learning how to breastfeed. What's that, you ask? Isn't breastfeeding the most natural thing in the world? Indeed, as natural as anything it takes weeks of exhausting work to figure out while leaving your boobs more tweaked than a meth addict.

That's right. I won't win any popularity contests here, but in spite of how sweet the bonding can really be from nursing your own precious child through her first months or years of life (not to mention through illness, teething, and a host of other ailments for which there is no better antidote), there are, it must be said, some things you should know about breastfeeding that may correlate with historical depictions of cartoon-like torture. Sure, nursing is an ideal method for feeding your child, even if you can only swing it for six weeks, during which most of the benefits are said to occur. But it is no great shakes while you're trying to figure it out.

"There are three reasons for breast-feeding: the milk is always at the right temperature; it comes in attractive containers; and the cat can't get it."

—Irena Chalmers

For many women, just getting to finally master this unique form of torture is a luxury, due to latching issues, problems with flow, how much milk you make, certain medications you may be taking, and so on. For those reasons, and a thousand others, you might consider formula feeding. Formula feeding is nourishing and convenient, because any reasonably capable human can give your baby a bottle. If that's the road you choose, great. Do what's best for you and your baby. If you encounter judgy interlopers who lecture you, tell them just that: your feeding plan works best for you and your baby. Period. End of conversation.

If you decide to give breastfeeding a go, however, there are some potential trouble spots you should know about up front. The first issue is that breastfeeding must be learned. By you *and* the baby. Though your baby is born with a rooting instinct to look for and suckle the breast, she has to learn to latch—a specific kind of mouth positioning and sucking that stimulates the breast to get your milk flowing and looks like your baby is about to mouth a cantaloupe. And you have to learn how to teach her how to do that. For many women, this requires days and weeks of trial and error when you happen to be at your most vulnerable, not to mention emotional. After one day of trying for what seemed like hours to get my baby to latch on and not just use me as a giant pacifier, I burst into tears, convinced I was a complete failure. I have heard from approximately 37 million women that they went through this exact same process.

Once it clicked, it clicked, and I went on to happily nurse my baby for two and a half years. I'm nothing if not an advocate, but I will never forget how miserable I felt for weeks until it all made sense. Those medieval Europeans had no idea that, if they really wanted to make women suffer, they could have just let them nurse their children untended. Cases in point:

. . .

The Heretic's Fork: Worn like a choker with a prod attached to it, featuring two sharp metal points under the chin and another two just below the collar bone (Google it), this little beauty greatly inhibited the wearer's ability to do much of anything but come clean about her witchery.

The Nursing Fork: Depending on your boob size, you may find yourself lying on your side or contorting in odd, scoliosis-inducing angles for half an hour at a time to get your baby in the right position for latching on. The larger the boobs, the better chance you can at least lie on your side to feed. Though it won't stop you from experiencing numb hands and tingling elbows for as long as you nurse.

. . .

The Boots: Legs were wrapped in any number of materials, then bound until immovable, then roasted or pulverized using a variety of exciting and awful techniques.

The Nursing Boots: It may seem like any chance to sit down is a good thing for a new mother, but not moving your legs for minutes on end will often feel like forced torture for those several times throughout the day when you are confined to a chair or bed while you figure out this latching thing, and your baby nurses for what seems like forever. No big deal unless you need to pee, or do some work, or make something to eat, or answer the door, or any number of things that will only come up while you are sitting there.

. . .

Sleep Deprivation: Self-explanatory forced inability to sleep by using light, noise, or other methods to keep someone awake.

Nursing Sleep Deprivation: Until you master the "dream feeding" technique of getting your baby on the breast without even waking up, you'll be wide-awake every four-to-six for what feels like eternity. This is happy, joyous hell.

. . .

The Interrogation Chair: A chair with tons of tiny little sharp points or spikes covering it, to make sitting for a long period of time painful.

The Nursing Chair: Best used in conjunction with the Nursing Boots. Get used to sitting in that chair for the next several months or years while you hash this thing out. If your baby is sick or hitting a growth spurt, you might nurse her twice as often throughout the day and evening. That's when the odd tingling starts, the cramping, the pains. As your body's internal organs have completely shifted, no amount of contorting makes it comfortable.

. . .

Thumbscrews: The thumbs were placed on wooden bars between screws that were slowly tightened to cause great pain.

Nursing Thumbscrews: Replace your thumbs with your nipples. Incorrect latching over multiple nursing sessions can leave your nipples chewed up, bleeding, and even *detached from the areola.* If this happens to you, you will know pain. Did I mention you have to keep nursing through it?

. . .

The Breast Ripper: This metal claw that was said to pierce the breast and shred it is even excruciating to consider.

The Nursing Breast Ripper: Also known as mastitis, a breast infection occurring from even one bad latch that breaks the skin and allows an infection to happen, it leaves you with flu-like feelings and one miserable, hot, stinging boob. Did I also mention that you must keep nursing with it? One of the worst pains I have ever endured. If it were be combined with Burning Vulva, I'd tell anyone everything.

. . .

The Inquisition: The repetitive form of torture involving questions asked over and over again until the victim would break.

The Nursing Inquisition: You'll nurse over and over again at first, to seemingly no effect, while your breasts swell and get hot, and you begin to sweat. A lactation consultant may be called in to question your every move, the size of your breasts, the errant positioning of your nipples, your shoddy technique. This all comes to a cruel, torturous head when you eventually realize your child was merely using you as a giant pacifier this whole time and wasn't even feeding. Back to square one! With your sore, tired, achy, protesting breasts.

. . .

Of course, it's not all for nothing. Eventually, those boobs are going to pull through. You will probably get the hang of it. And anyone who gets in the daily swing of nursing a baby knows that the prolactin— a.k.a. "Mommy Valium"—is the best friend you never knew you could have.

If it works for you, you'll have a sense of triumph that you really did this thing at a time when, historically, work and economics mean fewer women than ever can nurse at all, much less longer than a few weeks. And that is nothing to wince at.

ROCKING IT . . . YOUR LIFE WITH BABY

29.

THE GREAT BABY EXCUSE

Even though your new life with your baby means you're filled with a confusing mixture of awe-inspiring love and brutally sleepless nights, know this: You have your hand on the pull-cord of a terrific trapdoor. A golden baby parachute, if you will, crafted out of only the finest bamboo cloth diaper.

That's right: That baby of yours has just heralded in a new era of social and obligational freedom in your life. This is it! The time when you no longer have to do a bunch of stuff you hate with people you barely like, or what I called the Golden Years. You have found yourself in the possession of an excuse that only the most aggressive meddlers have the nerve to question: a baby.

That's right: If you are a bit misanthropic, a little shy, really reclusive, or merely a run-of-the-mill homebody, consider this kid your new one-stop excuse for avoiding all kinds of social hassles for years to come. You have all the guilt-free license in the world to crowd out everything, and everyone, that no longer fits in your life with baby.

Think of the possibilities! Your baby is a squishy, lovable, bulletproof reason to do and not do a million things you never even realized you wanted to do or not do in the first place. And anyone who suggests it's anything but so pure it floats gets the what-for of the century for being a big, jerk-faced family hater. Win-win-win-win to infinity. Times a billion.

So use your baby for the good opportunity she represents. (Also love her in a healthy way, duh, but feel free to take a little here, too, especially because she's more than happy to usurp your time!)

Here are some things your bundle of joy can help you get rid of:

» **Bad friends:** There's never been a better time to be "too busy" than when the friend you're not really friends with but who thinks you two are besties wants to come over and chat again about how her life isn't going so great and she really needs a pep talk from you.

» **Bad roommates:** You've had a baby! You can't live with someone who burns incense on the daily and smokes clove cigarettes inside. It's just not viable. Furthermore, did you want your baby to listen to house music? I didn't think so.

» **Bad acquaintances:** You can't even wave hello and chat for two seconds with that dude who always lingers for way too long because, HELLO, you're too busy making sure your baby doesn't stick a marble in her nose.

Your baby is an excellent excuse to get out of the following situations:

» **Office cocktail hour:** You can't drink anyway if you're nursing, so no more racking your brain for "believable" family entanglements.

» **Faking sick days:** Your baby is sick, like, constantly. That's what babies do at first. No more rehearsing the fatigue and light residual cough of faux-flu symptoms upon your return. Bonus sympathy if you actually get sick from your kid. That will happen more often than it won't.

» **Friday-night blockbuster with friend who has bad taste:** Don't want to watch *Brokedown Palace Part Two: Once a Mule, Always a Mule* in theaters? You just had a baby. And your baby really wants you to wait until it's out on Netflix.

If this seems like an embarrassment of riches, it's because it is. And there's even MORE good news: This get-out-of-jail-free card never expires. (Well, not for eighteen or so YEARS, so who's counting?)

But there's also bad news (sorry?), which I saved until last on purpose: Approximately 99 percent of the time you invoke a child-related excuse to avoid doing something "fun," you won't even be lying.

Yeah. See, that's the record-scratcher on this one. Sometimes said baby will actually cause you to miss things that are fun-fun, no ironic quote marks needed. (Those things are very, very rare, though, and for once in your life you will actually never regret missing anything if it allows you to get more sleep.)

Needless to say, the first few years of a baby's life are fraught with immune system–building scares. A fever here, a rash there, a cough that turns particularly juicy-sounding, and a runny nose that won't stop. If your baby is in the rotating germ feeder we call daycare, triple that. You knew this kinda—have you ever seen a young child *without* a runny nose?—and yet, you had no idea until it happened to you.

But the bad side has another upside: After all this isolated time in the trenches caring for your pod while she fashions an immune system, you will bow out of social obligations without so much as a faint smidge of guilt. You'll have earned it. Even when so-and-so can't understand why you don't want to come play beer pong at your old favorite dive bar.

To make this dodge easier, I offer a solid tip from the trenches: Print up a list of all the possible baby-related illnesses that can befall a young'un, cut them into strips, and put them in a hat to draw from whenever you need a good one. This way, they are random but realistic. Make sure to repeat reoccurring illnesses that are oh-so-common in infants, and use this to fill in the gaps between your honest excuses.

A sample list:

» Cold.
» Fever.
» Cold.

» Fever.
» Up all night with colic.
» Runny nose.
» Cough's gotten junky-sounding.
» Had a runny nose, but now she's got a high fever again.
» Cold.
» Up all night with baby who couldn't breathe through her nose.
» Tugging at her ears again—looks like another ear infection.
» Fussy baby.
» Double ear infection.
» Cold.
» Cold.
» Runny nose.
» Diaper rash.
» Fussy baby.

Seriously: A cold really can last for weeks for a baby. Fevers come and go like crazy ex-boyfriends at your favorite bar. If someone finds it odd that you used a double ear infection twice in one month as a reason to dodge yet another brutally un-fun office party where everyone stands around talking about *Two and a Half Men,* that's his problem. Let him go home and search the Internet on his own free time to discover that back-to-back double ear infections—especially in winter!—are super common in babies. Booyah! (Boohoo.)

30.

FOUR TYPES OF WOMEN WHEN IT COMES TO POST-BIRTH SEX

Unfathomably, while dealing with all the discomforts and tribulations of post-birth recovery, someone such as your husband, boyfriend, partner, or a total rando will want to get it on with you after you have a baby. This will happen *well* before it even occurred to you that you even could get it on. Is that even possible? Does that person know what went on down there?!

If it seemed like pregnancy itself was full of sticky-trap messages about what to care about and not care about, so is post-birth, when you are supposed to simultaneously heal your way into new motherhood and transform into a ferocious, MILFy kitten in the sack who has magically reinhabited your old vagina like a NSFW *Freaky Friday* version of *Body Snatchers.*

Did you know that even if you are zombie-tired and your vagina feels like a slinky that your number-one goal (after your other number-one goals of taking care of your baby, taking care of yourself, figuring out your career, and working on your communication with your partner) should be having sex with that partner as soon as possible?

But it's for a good reason: because having sex after the baby helps you heal quicker. Just kidding; it's because if you let your groove slip away for too long, it'll be out the door and down the street in your neighbor's bedroom before you can say "butt plug." D'oh!

As always, you'll turn to lady mags and Internet communities for comfort, where exactly zero of the pieces helping you navigate this steamy road will be titled "Take as Long as You Damn Well Please to Do It Again." Instead, they will be called things like "How to get Your Love Life Back" and "Six Ways to Steam Up Your Sex Life." You'll read about "How to Get Your Groove Back" and "How to Have Great Sex After Having a Baby!"

And always, with the finger-wagging refrain, get back to the doing and having of the sex as fast as possible, or else, sad trombone, your relationship is DOOMED FOREVER. Can you spell *divorce*? Does it have fewer letters than *lingerie*? You could be in trouble. Good thing loose-fitting jeans with an elastic waistband come in handy for being UTTERLY ALONE (with your baby).

But what none of this is helping any freshly birthed baby mama do is figure out how she actually feels about sex now. After all, you're the one with the slinky vagina, remember? Conventional wisdom is changing about when it's actually okay to have sex—typically, caregivers say six weeks is a solid bet, but more and more these days, they say after two weeks, or when the bleeding stops, you are okay to go. (Check, as always, with your doctor.) But assuming your equipment is in mint condish, whether you actually want to get to cuddling after the mind-numbing work of caring for a newborn is and should be the biggest determining factor in how to proceed down the tenuous path of doin' the dirty post-baby. Here are the four types of women you might see in the mirror when it comes to post-birth sex.

Hot and Cold

Like being stuck in the throes of menopausal madness, you don't know if you're coming (ha! You're definitely not coming) or going. One minute you want your partner all over you like white on rice, and the next minute you would be totally cool if he disappeared forever into the bowels of hell. Freezing hell. This may sound like an agonizing place to be in, and it no doubt is, to say nothing of how maddening it is to try to schedule sex in this condition, but at least it means you've still got the fire rumbling in there somewhere—it's just unregulated.

Protip: When you feel the heat rising at an opportune moment, go with it. Don't talk yourself out of it on account of it being late, or you being tired, or there always being laundry to fold. Announce that business is open and your partner better get it while the getting is good. That technique has the added benefit of a sense of spontaneity, but allows you to retain the control you need over when and how this goes down.

Hot Hot Hot

You're on, you're on, you're on, and you're never off. If somehow you've been blessed with being horny as hell now that this baby is out of you, you don't need my help; you need to help me. And others.

Protip: Become a sex surrogate? Shut up already?

Cold as Ice

If you're as cold as a Foreigner song in Alaska and the idea of sex makes you want to crawl back into your own vagina for the winter, then you should take as long as you damn well please to get uncomfortably back on this horse. If that time becomes longer than, say, three months, then I think you should consider why, but you should allow yourself another two months to do it. Then, if you still can't shake it, see a doctor, but only begrudgingly, and never at the one time you could be napping.

Protip: If you're just going to drop out of doing it altogether for nearly half a year, I suggest being an intoxicating conversationalist. In lieu of that, try handjobs. Even a poorly done one will get the job done, and you'll still have one hand free to do laundry.

Warm and Frightened

I'm willing to bet that lots of women would like to have sex again a few weeks after childbirth but are uncertain about how it will feel, or what their bodies will be like, or if they will just fall asleep, or worse, if their husbands will just fall asleep. It's certainly how I felt, so it must be the norm! But really, if you are into the idea but you're just not the most confident sexual being in the universe, rest assured lots of ladies are in postpartum purgatory with you.

For one, the fears about sex feeling weird or off are not unfounded. The first time I had a penis inside me again I was sure that penis was comprised of a series of steel cubes. It wasn't cold but it felt like either it or my vagina was comprised of quadrants, and I could feel things in places I didn't remember feeling them before—or had I really been that drunk all those times?

Furthermore, everything wasn't as instantly lubed-up as it had been, and this made the steel-cube effect even more pronounced. Additionally, because of everything I was going through in this funhouse of quadrants and cubes, I felt compelled to narrate the entire experience for my husband. He'll accept your sympathy letters.

Protip: It gets better. Within a few weeks, things returned to normal and sex was no longer a cube-y, quadrant-y terror but rather as good as new again. In some ways, actually better. What they say about the closeness of experiencing childbirth with someone you love and how that can turn up the heat in the bedroom is super true, even if you're working with one super-heated-up cube at first.

31.

HOW TO BE COOL
WITH A BABY

You used to be one cool customer, you're probably thinking right about now. And then you had a baby and pushed out all traces of cool along with your placenta. (Fine print: Eating the placenta does not guarantee retaining said coolness.) Still, you don't have to throw the cool baby out with the cool bathwater. It is possible to both be a mother and be cool, in spite of what your brain and mirrors might tell you.

But like figuring out the exact right backdoor formula to get your kid into the best charter school in town, cool is elusive. Like determining whether that chick you stand next to at barre class who is sometimes nice but sometimes a hosebeast is actually your friend, cool is whimsical. Like trying to pin down exactly which low-rise jeans signal to the world that you're older now, but you haven't completely given up and are not a complete jackal, cool is unpredictable. And like discovering the exact reason why it has to burn so much when you pee after giving birth, cool is mysterious.

But it isn't rocket science. It literally isn't. It may not be easy to be cool, but it certainly shouldn't be extremely hard either. That's the contradictory nature of cool: It is, at its core, the result of two competing ideas: contrived effortlessness. All you have to do is make just enough of an effort to seem like you don't care. (Bonus points if you really, truly don't care—the holy grail of cool.)

I know a thing or two about cool because I was a music critic for five years. I watched bands every night. I took shots with rock stars (sorta). I stayed up late and got records for free and had very, very, very interesting conversations about how quickly a chorus should start in a truly catchy pop song.

During this time, after much trial and tribulation, I learned how to call cool in a matter of seconds. Even if I couldn't always articulate what made this band of four guys in white T-shirts and jeans hella cool while this other band with four guys in white T-shirts and jeans were lamecakes, I knew right away whether someone cut the cool mustard. (No truly cool person has ever said that.)

Then I had a baby. And the first thing I wanted to never do was step so much as one foot inside a rock club. The last thing I wanted to do was sit around debating the merits of whether such-and-such noisy garage band was the good kind of derivative or the bad kind, or the kind that makes you want to stab someone. I especially did not want to do this anywhere near the vicinity of a whiff of whisky, which now seemed repulsive.

What the hell had changed? In the face of making actual, breathing life, everything that seemed even remotely cool to me prior now suddenly seemed false. Lame. Desperate. Out of touch. The ultimate pose.

In part, it was because, suddenly, here I was with a living person who had brought with her a torrential downpour of emotion. I'd had to rethink my life and existence and entire perspective to welcome her into my life. This had made me happier, healthier, and totally into my new mission. But I was also on tenuous identity-ground, unsure of how to be my old self and still be this new person who suddenly cared a lot. What could be less cool than that?

"When you're pregnant, you can think of nothing but having your own body to yourself again; yet after having given birth you realize that the biggest part of you is now somehow external, subject to all sorts of dangers and disappearance, so you spend the rest of your life trying to figure out how to keep her close enough for comfort. That's the strange thing about being a mother: Until you have a baby, you don't even realize how much you were missing one."

—Jodi Picoult, *Vanishing Acts*

Was it even possible to be cool while actually caring about something besides yourself so much that you don't give a shit what anyone thinks about you? Could you do this while literally being the most tired you'd ever been in your entire life?

Actually, yes. In fact, I think I had it all wrong in the first place, and that's what cool actually is: caring about something that's not you. It reminds me of what White Stripes singer Jack White once said about why he had to escape the Detroit rock scene: he was no longer interested in navigating the minefield of cool, constantly having to prove by getting this reference or that that he was still cool. But, of course, not caring about the riffraff of the cool wars made Jack White infinitely more elusive, more unpredictable, and therefore cooler than ever.

In other words, being cool isn't about not caring about anything. It's about not caring about being cool. That said, you, as a new mom finding your way, are still on the precipice here, and remaining cool, which I just use as a shorthand for staying interesting, is one more thing you'll have to do now, like exercising or pumping breast milk. But the cool thing about cool is that it has a lot of built-in shortcuts. And all your cool doesn't really disappear with childbirth.

That said, if you want to make sure it doesn't entirely slip away, you'll need the following items:

» A sense of humor.
» Caffeine.
» Ibuprofen.
» Magazines.
» Internet.
» Television.

Once armed with these things, you can face and overcome the following challenges to your coolness.

. . .

The Challenge: You only care about baby stuff.

The Solution: Motherhood is, by definition, caring about baby stuff. It is also but one part of your new life. It will, no doubt, consume the majority of your waking thoughts at first, and will influence the choices you make for a lifetime, double no doubt. If it doesn't, something is fucked up and cool won't fix it. But this doesn't mean that everything else you were ever into has now been drop-shipped into a cryogenic vat. You still like vintage British cars and David Sedaris essays and old episodes of *My So-Called Life*. You still want to invent something. You still like fake absinthe. You're still in there, somewhere!

If you find yourself in a sinkhole of baby-think, flip the script. Pick something you used to spend loads of time thinking about that has nothing whatsoever to do with babies, and swill it around and reacquaint yourself with its textures. It will come back to you, bit by bit, piece by piece, utterance by utterance.

. . .

The Challenge: Everything maternal feels so earnest and heartfelt and threatens to swallow you whole.

The Solution: Motherhood is nothing if not a sappy Lifetime movie replete with tenderly played strings and gauzy nostalgia. But not all mothers toss on a floral jumper and head to the rocking chair. Try reading/viewing/absorbing the work of cool mothers you admire: Take in some essays from fascinating mothers such as Joan Didion or Patti Smith when you have a minute to spare. Dive into the poetry of frustrated housewife Anne Sexton. Steep when you can in the concerns of the tirelessly interesting mother, and you will see that for many women, having children no doubt influenced their brainscapes but never truly altered their original passions or interests. The old you may grow more distant by the diaper change, but the life of the mind is a tough thing to destroy in just one major vaginal push. It'll keep.

. . .

The Challenge: You've fallen in a baby hole and can't get out.

Solution: Remember that scene in *Poltergeist* where they tie a rope around the mom's waist and toss her into another dimension to go find her daughter? This is what I picture when you're in the baby hole, that no-man's land of lost souls where a mother can no longer speak full sentences or comprehend the concerns of adults. The only solution is to make someone yank the cord and pull you back into reality. Do this by reading something in any one of your nonbaby areas of interest for five minutes every day.

I know, I know, so many mommy lifestyle pieces will annoyingly suggest that you "carve out me-time" or "schedule a date . . . with yourself." I'm not going to insult you. I know that even if you somehow find two free hours during those first several months of new motherhood, the closest thing to a date with yourself probably means popping a vat of painkillers and catching up on reality TV. You'll hardly feel like using what rare time you get to reacquaint yourself with local politics. But stay with me here. I'm saying literally spend five minutes and only five minutes scanning a piece of longform journalism on a subject you care about, looking at a slideshow of interesting couture, or browsing a blog about politics. You'd be amazed what you can retain from only five minutes of Internet browsing and how it will come back to you in dire moments of soul-sucking boredom while you try to convince an infant to sleep. It's more than enough to stay current and of the world you were in, which is a cornerstone of being interesting, relevant, and yes, cool.

. . .

The Challenge: You're humorless.

The Solution: You're talking to someone who could get so hungry while breastfeeding that she could fly into a fit of sobs if the meatloaf wasn't warm enough. If you cannot laugh at raging meatloaf monster-face, you are fucked. Force yourself to see the humor in the crushing isolation of new motherhood. When you're dead-tired, lonely as hell while your husband works fifteen hours a day, and having none of it, try forcing your brain to tell this story of yours to someone else, only make it funny.

For me, that meant imagining that I was starring in a terrible sitcom about the clichés of pregnancy on loop, with every fart joke, unpredictable sob, and angry ravaging of another helpless plate of food. It was too cliché to be upset about it. And I found myself laughing at myself, and also at really bad television (*My Wife and Kids*, anyone?). I still really can't believe that someone who used to have what I considered a discerning sense of humor was now cracking up at *Two and a Half Men* and *Everybody Loves Raymond*. Not cool? The catch was, I didn't give two and a half shits. The joke was me, and that was actually pretty liberating.

. . .

The Challenge: You can barely hold a conversation that doesn't revolve around naps, feedings, or the merits of letting your baby cry it out.

The Solution: Remember how you made conversation before you had a baby? Where you talked about something in the news or a piece of art or a book you'd read? Do that again. Look, you had a baby; you didn't have a lobotomy. Although it totally feels that way because it probably is chemically or medically true, it's not true-true. Like, not forever-true. Truth. If, by the grace of God, you can actually interact with other humans, consider yourself super lucky. Spend a few minutes regaling these friends with the joys and horrors of parenting, but only the really funny ones. And then, change the subject. To them. To wallpaper. To anything. This seems obvious, and yet tons of new mothers blather on and on about the baby situation as if it's never happened to anyone before them and as if everyone else is dying to hear about the challenges of cloth diapers. Have mercy on those around you; win cool points forever.

. . .

In conclusion, by simply making the tiniest effort to cultivate interest in subjects outside of the deadeningly boring talk of babies, you will remain the cool person you were. If you have the time or wherewithal to work on a project, keep making art, take up a hobby, or do anything other than just be a caregiver, you're already an advanced cool person. But make no mistake: Caring about your baby and wanting the best for her are not lame. And you should never feel like these subjects are too uncool to bring up. Anyone who makes you feel that way isn't worth impressing. Still, if I may make one final plea: Do not, under any circumstances, start a mom-rap group. That is as lame as it gets.

32.

BEING A MOM ISN'T EASY—YOU'LL NEED A LITTLE HELP FROM YOUR "FRIENDS"

If you'd been born even a half-century ago, you'd be more likely to have a group of women around you to lend a helping hand—mothers, grandmothers, aunts, sisters, in-laws—and a relative uniformity in approach. Today, you might live all the way across the country, not talk to your family that much, or prefer hiring a pit bull over your own relatives to help you raise your children.

No matter. You can assemble your own team of expert caregivers to crowdsource for wisdom and hand-me-downs. Think of them as your very own Dirty Dozen. No, I'm not talking about your team of convicts to martyr yourself with against the Germans in a mass-assassination mission, but more like a crew of as many army buddies as you can rally consisting of other moms (or dads) who can help you navigate this tricky new time in your life.

There are as many kinds of parents as there are parenting methods, and each of them can offer some guidance as you navigate this precarious path, from the Morally Superior Mom to the Hyper-Fun Mom to the

Health-Nut Mom. They all offer a good tip for the trenches, and on occasion, they come with the added benefit of actual friendship.

You can find these people at playgrounds, at daycare, at the pediatrician's office. On Facebook mom groups, on message boards. Anywhere there's a place to talk about the actual best salve-to-ass ratio on a newborn is a built-in crew of ladies worth recruiting. Such as:

The Morally Superior Mom

This mother is a smug pain in your ass, to say nothing of her children's asses, but her running superior commentary on the lives and choices of all other mothers is actually really useful. As she details the ways in which other mothers are nowhere near up to snuff because they expose their children to Disney, BPA, the wrong kinds of diapers, or any diapers at all, keep in mind that checking in with this lady every so often is actually efficient. Think of her as your one-stop shop for the issues of the day. Whatever women are stewing about on the parenting front—the cost of a nanny, the best charter school in town, the immunization schedule—she'll keep you abreast of the issues and save you all the trouble of crafting the arguments. Use her. Mine her. Just let her keep all the anxiety to herself.

The Hyper-Fun Mom, a.k.a. the Soak-Off

While fun, this mother can also be through-the-roof up on your nerves or the source of your greatest insecurities about being a super cool mother. She bursts into song midsentence. She's like Jim Carrey and Robin Williams doing caricatures of themselves in tandem, on steroids, only scarier. She is almost totally impossible to even associate with. But think of her as the military equivalent of the soak-off: someone you send out to absorb the first round of heat to buy time.

And oddly enough, kids love her. She never, ever misses an opportunity to round up the nearby children for a game of choo-choo. If you ever needed a mom who will take all the work of entertaining your children on herself, it's this lady. She's a clown, an art teacher, a music teacher, and a general entertainer all rolled into one. Call her when you don't feel like getting off the couch.

The Health-Nut Mom

It's important to have a standard, and extreme moms always help you gauge exactly how lax you've been with your own kid. The Health-Nut Mom might seem intimidating or boorish, but she's actually a great way to keep perspective about exactly how far down the road of processed foods you've gotten, to say nothing of her value when trying to figure out which veggie sausage is the most likely to go down your kid's gullet with the least griping.

After all, you DO actually care a lot about feeding your child a healthy diet, just not enough to replace all fun foods with mashed yeast. Health-Nut Mom always has a good granola recipe! She will also probably help you keep a running commentary of every errant edible, and along with her tallying you can keep your own considerably more chilled-out score. Sure, you let your kid have that lollipop, but you also made sure she had blueberries and broccoli, and you spent one-eighth of the time freaking out. She's also the best mom-house to drop your kids off at for an afternoon, because you know they won't be returned to you vibrating with sugar.

The Affluent Mom

She has a nanny, her kids have the best bedding from Pottery Barn Kids and top-notch super-expensive toys, she throws the best birthday parties, and she buys all the best organic snacks. Affluent Moms are the easiest to hate reflexively, but hating her would mean missing out on the fact that she's a great goalpost for figuring out what, exactly, you are allegedly aspiring to. Is the rat race worth it? Is she really any happier? Do you actually give a shit about stroller brands? Nope. And yet, my lack of good breeding meant I had no clue what kind of fancy school I was supposed to covet for my daughter. I luckily made a friend who knew all the right schools, not to mention all the right methods, for getting into them.

I picked her brain and it helped me pare down an argument I would have had in a vacuum in my own head for the rest of my life: exactly what blend of public and private schools I'd want—and be able and willing to pay for—when my daughter hits kindergarten. Likewise with toys. Getting to see the top-of-the-line, spare-no-expense kind of playroom lets you modify your own game plan within your budget. Does your kid really need every single item from the Pottery Barn Kids retro kitchen suite? Nah. Especially not when she can play with it at Affluent Mom's house!

The Chill Mom

This mom could not be more laid back if she were roastin' a blunt at the playground. Maybe it's the antidepressants, or maybe she's just that cool, but either way, nothing gets to this woman. She's chill, her husband is chill, and their kid is pretty chill, for a kid. Hanging out with them not only helps you relax, but it makes you realize that no matter what you're sweating, it's probably not worth going on the warpath, disrupting the daily routine, or actually raising your voice about. Relax. Let it ride.

The Nutbag

How this woman ever got to be a mom is beyond you (welcome to the other side of judgy-ness!), but it's definitely worth checking in with her every now and again (by phone! Never in person!) to remind yourself what rock bottom looks like. I'm not talking about harsh judgment or mockery. I'm talking about genuine concern for her and her children's well-being that also happens to provide you with the added benefit of a real-life illustration of everything you are happy didn't happen to you (by phone).

A regular mom would score some painkillers from a friend who just had her wisdom teeth out to relax on a Friday night. Nutbag Mom fakes the prescription, gets busted, does a few years in jail, gets busted again, and does a few more years. All the while, her kid is raised by her grandmother, and did I mention you have never been happier to only be able to take half a painkiller at a time anyway? This is the mom to talk to (by phone!) when you think you fucked up by forgetting to turn in your kid's preschool application. Feeling crappy? You won't when she mentions that she missed her probation meeting—again.

The Beta Mom

The Beta Mom is not a bad mom. She loves her kid like crazy. She'd do anything for him. Well, not *anything*, heh. She's not going to take a week off to potty train him or actually worry too much about homework, or planning stuff, or getting caught up in the craziness of all the competition. Did she tell you about the time she took a shower, got out, and realized her kid had finally learned to let himself out the front door? She found him fifteen minutes later playing with friends six houses down the block.

Weirdly, her kid turns out just as smart and interesting and lovable as everyone else's, not in spite of the fact that she doesn't care about all that shit, but because she doesn't. She makes up for what she lacks in the June Cleaver department with old-fashioned, organic love. This mom is always good for a laugh and a reminder not to sweat the small stuff but to still do the big stuff. Mistakes happen. Have a glass of wine and a (legally obtained) painkiller, and don't overthink it.

Germaphobe Mom

Did you know there were germs? Of course you did. So does she. In fact, it's all she ever thinks about. Sometimes when she's just trying to relax all she can think about is all the stuff all over all the remotes that she forgot to sanitize immediately after use this morning. This mom is great for having hand sanitizer at the playground. Oftentimes she can be seen pulling up in a fire truck filled completely with hand sanitizer to hose the entire place down, just in case. She's also good for reminding you to wash your hands when everyone is coming down with the flu, but she is literally not useful to you for much else. Well, I guess if things are going too well and you need some needless anxiety in your life, give her a call.

The Single Mom

Many married women dread the Single Mom, because they fear she will either show them up with her single-handed parenting chops or steal their husbands and refashion them for herself. This is nonsense. The Single Mom is there to commiserate when you're stuck with the baby by yourself, and to remind you that you can totally do this. And if she's a single *party* mom, double the fun. She can never bring too much wine to the get-together, and she's the first to admit that she will be waking up the next morning, turning on the cartoons, and going straight back to bed.

The Hyper-Organized Mom

You need a mom-friend who will collect the money for the big present for the daycare provider. Who will organize the playdates for the kids who are really good friends at the preschool. Who will notice which kids are really good friends at the preschool. Who will help with the birthday party you forgot to plan for the kids at the preschool.

The Super Touchy-Feely Mom

Not to be confused with the Health-Nut Mom, the Super Touchy-Feely Mom is so comfortable with feelings, and talking about feelings, and good vibes, and positive settings, that she's just uplifting to be around. She's good to just let it all out, vibe it all up, and keep it on the sunny side.

The Crafty Mom

Somebody found Pinterest, and somebody has about a bajillion ideas for a rainy day. Wanna make superhero costumes for Halloween? A fairy house out of stuff you find in the yard? Six great recipes for funny-faced cookies your kids can help with? Born to homeschool, the Crafty Mom will do all the work and needs none of the credit for providing you with tip upon tip for how to enhance your baby's life with nonstop activity. She's great for calling the night before the Valentine's Day party when you need an idea for the homemade cards. You weren't considering *store-bought* ones, were you!?

The Fix-It Dad

If you want to be around the people who are typically culturally groomed to never freak out in the face of injury or blood, Fix-It Dads are your best bet. They know how to DO stuff. Stuff you didn't feel like learning to do, like fashioning a bandage out of a tampon. They are excellent backup on the playground. They can fix errant stroller wheels. They can repair the baby gate that's coming off the wall, etc.

. . .

While all of us have a little bit of all these parenting types in us, it never hurts to have an expert or a varied approach to the hot mess that is watching a baby like a hawk. And never forget: if you combine powers, you'll never meet a parenting mission you can't sail through.

33.

ALL BABIES ARE SWEET, PRECIOUS BUNDLES OF JOY, AND OTHER BABY MYTHS

When people talk about babies, they tend to talk in extremes, and for good reason: The extremes really are extreme. Motherhood and infancy are either a blissful path to enlightenment or a dive off a razor-edged cliff directly into the mouth of the hellbeast. It's a wonderful, life-affirming time here to finally complete you, Jerry Maguire–style, or it's *Rosemary's Baby*. What people tend to forget to mention is that sometimes you'd be more than willing to settle for Rosemary's baby if only it meant you had the time, money, and self-confidence to still pull off a pixie cut.

While we're on the subject of movies starring Tom Cruise, I have never wanted to be the sort of person who would quote *Vanilla Sky*, but here goes: "Because without the bitter baby, the sweet ain't as sweet." Still there? Whew.

I knew that was going to be a tough sell. But it's true: Raising a small child can be both soul-filling and soul-deadening, what I like to think of as a bucolic nightmare. Sometimes it will no doubt feel like full-on bucolic plague. But when everything is running exactly as it should be, you can be filled with pleasant contentment or even utter joy while simultaneously filled with despair-inducing shell-shock. Sometimes they flip. Sometimes they flop.

"Raising kids is part joy and part guerrilla warfare."

—Ed Asner

For the unplanned pregnancy–haver, it is, I submit, even harder to hoe these poopy rows, because this knowledge is no doubt what made you so baby-averse in the first place. But what you weren't counting on was the fact that, just like Mia Farrow in *Rosemary's Baby*, you'll find yourself pushing that stroller happily along no matter how much your child, exhausted from fighting her nap and tired from still not having learned how to latch on correctly to nurse, reminds you of Satan's spawn. .

You'll still be utterly ecstatic to get to know her, even when she is literally punching you in the face or biting you on the shoulder. Of course, note that I didn't say anywhere in here that you wouldn't still be annoyed. You will still definitely always totally have the energy to be pissed about that. Funny thing.

But in case you're too afraid to realize that right now while staring down at this very dependent, challenging blob, take heart: Nothing's ever all one way, all the time, and the rampant misconceptions about how babies are or are not don't really help much, though there's a nugget to truth in all of them. Such as:

The Myth: Babies never stop crying. Oh, really? Because they do, actually. They do stop. It's just that they start back up again much sooner than makes any sense considering everything you just did to get them to stop. This is not helped by the enormous number of reasons your baby could be crying in the first place that you have to decipher without anything like a baby Rosetta Stone. It can go beyond hunger, sleepiness, overstimulation, gas, an allergy to something, or an itchy tag and well into existential crisis. Babies just cry.

The Truth: Babies don't cry *that* much. Because no matter how much she cries, your baby really doesn't cry as much as you think. (Unless she's colicky, and then she really does cry for six hours straight. Ouch.) The problem is that one minute of real-time crying *feels like* twenty minutes. If you actually look at the clock, your baby is probably crying less than you think.

. . .

The Myth: Babies have to be held every single second. Do you like Velcro? Because you sorta just gave birth to some. Babies do need to be held almost constantly. Like, whatever is just a hair under constantly is exactly how much it's going to take here. Get used to that. That said, it's not technically constantly! But if you suspect you haven't been holding your baby all that much the last hour, pick her up. She's about to start crying her head off anyway. Try to beat her to the cry-punch.

The Truth: You can totally set your baby down long enough to read a magazine or watch a show. You absolutely can; anyone who says you can't is lying. The only time you can't is when you absolutely desperately need it the most or you'll drive off a cliff. That's when it will never happen. Count on it.

. . .

The Myth: Your body will be totally different after giving birth. In some ways, it will. It will be wrecked. Things inside will feel like they moved around to other weird places like a snowglobe, because they did. Your vagina will seem way more open for business than it ever did before, and by open for business I mean literally bigger. And wider. Your stomach is going to be like a pillowcase with no padding, and your vulva, well, let's just say you won't even realize you have one, if you ever did. It probably took off with your placenta.

The Truth: Your body will still mostly be like how it was before. But the funny thing is, your body is basically the same. It's still your body, the one you've known and loved. In spite of how insane-trashed it feels, it will soon be more like it used to be than like it is. If that makes sense. Believe me, it makes sense.

. . .

The Myth: Babies are maddeningly complex little buggers and impossible to figure out. Is she tired or does she just hate living rooms with orange couches? Is it the green and brown nursery theme she's protesting or your insistence on playing the Pixies on Saturday morning? Nothing about caring for a baby made any immediate sense to me, either intuitively or quickly. The only super easy thing was loving her. If I could have gotten a T-shirt from the hospital that said "I Swear, My Intentions Are Really Good" I would have worn it. Because that's literally all I came equipped with for taking care of my own infant. Okay, so I had arms and boobs, too, but I had to guess at how both of those would work with a baby.

The Truth: In some ways, babies are super easy to take care of. You get to know your baby pretty quickly, and she makes sense sooner than you think. She cries when you hold her awkwardly, and you realize that you were actually holding her like you might hold a jellyfish that just crapped on you. And mostly, she just wants to be with you.

. . .

The Myth: Babies are a total drag. Man, she does not think your commentary on the *90210* spinoff is particularly insightful. And she hates the organic strained peas.

The Truth: Babies are so much fun! You can put a pair of sunglasses on your baby and laugh for approximately three hours.

. . .

The Myth: Babies are a one-way ticket to utter reclusion. Sure, there will be times when that's the case, such as that few-month stage where she cries nonstop the SECOND the car-seat buckle touches her skin and for the duration of any trip. But the rest of the time, she probably doesn't mind the car.

The Truth: Babies can go anywhere. And yet when you toss her in a sling and board a plane, she's takes it like a champ.

. . .

The Myth: Babies are super boring. They *are* blobby blobs that mostly lie around doing the three Ps: peeing, pooping, and protesting. And you have to bear witness to every excruciating non-moment of it. But to YOU, those things are interesting.

The Truth: Babies are utterly fascinating. In retrospect, her every move and utterance was chock-full of all the personality she would one day express with words; I was just too exhausted and inexperienced to see it.

34.

REFLECTIONS

Once upon a time in the not-so-distant past, you were a newly pregnant, gobsmacked lady with no idea what to do when you found yourself knocked up. Could you ever survive it? What would you be like as a mother? Would you still have a partner at the end of the day, any friends, a life you could call your own, or at least the chance to finish reading anything longer than a tweet?

Here you are a year later, and if you're reading this, it's safe to assume the answer is yes. Maybe you even nailed it. Sure, it probably looks nothing like you imagined; it never does. But either way, it has been one wonderfully rocky road. You've no doubt learned some things about what you're capable of. I bet you even kind of know what you're doing now, or at least you no longer feel like an impostor in a foreign land of people who seem utterly at ease with parenting while you pretend to get it.

You are finally, at long last, no longer a crazy, shell-shocked person who has no idea what the hell is going on. I bet you've had some seriously crazy moments, often at 3:45 in the morning, and some seriously heartwarming ones that still catch you off-guard. I bet you've never felt more frightened and more capable at the same time. And though your body may finally feel like it did before (kinda), you're probably still farting in a weird way that sounds like clapping.

But you owe yourself a pretty big pat on the back. You are raising a baby even though you felt like the least qualified person in the universe to do it. That's amazing! It's also not that amazing. Because you were going to pull through, you know? You just had to figure it out.

"Whether your pregnancy was meticulously planned, medically coaxed, or happened by surprise, one thing is certain— your life will never be the same."

—Catherine Jones

Now that you have your sea legs, you can look around and take stock of a few things you were probably way too freaked out to even notice about the world of parenting. Like, have you noticed that:

» Other moms are just as freaked out as you are?
» You can spot a new mother a mile away?
» You can now identify when your baby needs to poop, has pooped, wants to poop, or is just pretending to poop?
» You can nurse or bottle-feed like a complete champ?
» Your vagina is almost like a vagina you used to know and even liked once? And that you kind of like how it's not exactly the same vagina anyway, almost as if you're getting to be two different women in one lifetime?
» You love the people who love you even more now that you've loved this child with them? And that you love even less the people

who had no interest in still being your friends during this journey? And that you're totally okay with that?

» Cloth or plastic, breast or bottle, attachment or shitty, that the main thing your baby needs is your love and attention, and none of that other shit matters all that much as long as you get him/her vaccinated? Just kidding—have you noticed that even the word *vaccine* raises your blood pressure now?

» Everything you think you know about your kid changes every few weeks, and that you can even tell when he/she's having growth spurts, milestone days, big brain changes, because suddenly now he/she's repeating what you said, or noticing what you're looking at, or walking more gracefully, or any number of things, and it never stops being really wild? Also, that everything—literally everything—is a choking hazard?

» Your exhaustion feels worth it at least 80 percent of the time?

» You've been forced to step outside yourself and consider someone else more important than yourself, and that these growing pains have been obnoxiously helpful and enlightening? But that you're still you in there, and in many ways, a better, more focused you? And a definitely more grown-up you? Possibly a you with an unimaginably greater capacity for compassion? Because there's literally more of you now?

» You are constantly in awe of what you were capable of doing with your body and soul, even though you are the sort of person who thinks that pretty much any sentence about a soul is super cheesy, and that you fed your soul without even meaning to?

I also bet that:

» You can get your baby back to sleep most nights.

» You have your own entire system for how to take all the weird, random shit you need with you to the park—and most days, you don't even forget to actually take it.

- » Instead of feeling like your happy accident was a lark or an embarrassment, your unplanned pregnancy is just another funny story among many to tell about the time you went jet-skiing at the lake and came back knocked up.
- » You would do this all over again, even if someone could have stopped you and told you how hard it would all be.
- » There was a time when you were the most frustrated, confused, mixed-up person in the universe, and now you are only as frustrated, confused, and mixed-up as everyone else.

"I came to parenting the way most of us do—knowing nothing and trying to learn everything."

—Mayim Bialik

I was reading a list recently of ten things you wish you'd known before coming a parent. It was everything I could now relate to: that those first few months are torturous, that you will go crazy over lack of sleep, that you don't need all that baby stuff you thought you did, that nothing will ever be the same. What struck me was that the list was relatable as all get-out, except for number one: making a baby isn't as easy at it sounds.

Which made me realize: After a certain length of time, your concerns are identical to that of any parent. You are no longer one of the 49 percent who had a baby unexpectedly. You're every parent who has ever had a kid and was changed by that kid as much or more than you are changing it (literally). And instead of feeling so different, weird, marginalized, and terrified like you might have while pregnant, you're now just as much of a zombie, sucker, hero, martyr, asshole, loving, caring, self-sacrificing parent as everyone else who does this. Congratulations! No question mark.

Which can only mean one thing: You're probably actually ready to have another one. Just kidding. Let's not get too carried away.

APPENDIX:

RESOURCES

A handful of books and websites were my go-to on pregnancy and childbirth and the first year of motherhood. These really resonated with me in tone and style.

Books

Keep in mind you'll probably get a dozen hand-me-down advice books from others, and they all have something or other worth remembering. You'll figure out what works for you, but until then, feel free to peruse lots of books until you hit one, or a hybrid of several, that makes sense. Some people never read the books at all and are totally cool, but that was not possible for me.

Gaskin, Ina May. *Ina May's Guide to Breastfeeding.* (New York, NY: Bantam Dell, 2009).
Ina May Gaskin is a birthing badass, a midwife who runs a commune in rural Tennessee and singlehandedly challenged the national C-section rate with her proven ability to deliver all kinds of babies from all kinds of vaginas. If you need a boost about what your body is capable of, you will get it in spades here.
Gaskin, Ina May. *Ina May's Guide to Childbirth.* (New York, NY: Bantam Dell, 2003).

Iovine, Vicki. *The Girlfriends' Guide to Pregnancy.* (New York, NY: Pocket Books, 1995, 2007).
A must-have to parse the highlights and horrors of pregnancy in a conversational tone.

Karp, Harvey. *The Happiest Baby on the Block.* (New York, NY: Bantam Dell, 2002).
A must for frustrated new parents struggling to calm, comfort, and soothe a little one, especially to sleep. It might not work for you, but these tricks are probably a necessary trial on your path to enlightenment with your particular child.

Murkoff, Heidi and Sharon Mazel. *What to Expect When You're Expecting.* (New York, NY: Workman Publishing Company, 1984, 1988, 1991, 1996, 2002, 2008).

It's unavoidable, but this compendium of chirpy-chanty pregnancy experiences is a great reference, and exhaustive. Just keep in mind that it's an uplifting experience and may not be the best outlet when you want to vent about how fat your ass feels.

Sears, William and Martha Sears. *The Attachment Parenting Book: A Commonsense Guide to Understanding and Nurturing Your Baby.* (New York, NY: Little, Brown and Company, 2001).

A very intuitive-feeling guide to raising a baby with lots of comfort and love.

Wolf, Naomi. *Misconceptions: Truth, Lies, and the Unexpected on the Journey to Motherhood.* (New York, NY: Anchor Books, 2003).

This book most helped me navigate the medical maze for pregnant women. Large portions of it seemed to appear directly from my head onto the page when it came to how it felt to be poked, prodded, and ushered through the labyrinth.

Websites

These websites were reputable references:

» American Academy of Pediatrics: *www.aap.org*
» American Pregnancy Association: *www.americanpregnancy.org* (pregnancy help)
» Ask Dr. Sears: *www.Askdrsears.com* (baby advice)
» KellyMom: *www.kellymom.com* (breastfeeding and weaning help)

ACKNOWLEDGMENTS

Thanks to my agent, Natasha Alexis, and editors, Halli Melnitsky and Laura Daly, for guiding me so assuredly through a bewilderingly large number of sentences. Thanks to Jezebel.com editor Jessica Coen, who took a chance on an unknown writer and gave me a weekly column. Thanks to the friends who put up with me while I was insufferably pregnant, weirdly emotional, and smelled like chicken-noodle soup, and yet still wanted to talk about, hear about, or give feedback on this experience/book: Adam Gold, Elizabeth Jones, Alexis Bartley Paulson, Jack Silverman, Jim Ridley, Patrick Rodgers, Caleb Hannan, P.J. Tobia, Ashley Spurgeon. Thanks to my former newspaper editor, Jim Ridley, who taught me the rhythm of good words, and Pete Kotz, who taught me how to sizzle them (and who also told me to have one hell of a baby, because, duh, babies are America). Thanks to my fancy Hollywood writing partner, Daisy Gardner, who listened to me ramble on and on about my preciously individual pregnant experience while she had two young children and could have easily bitched for twice as long.

And thanks to my husband, Lance, for sticking around gallantly through all of this, even though I once sobbed because the meatloaf he made me wasn't hot enough. Okay, twice. And to my sweet, hilarious Edie, my raison d'etre: I would be surprise-pregnant with you a thousand times again, no matter how fat I got.

INDEX

A

Alcohol, drinking,
25–30, 69–70, 76
Armstrong, Lance, 49
Asner, Ed, 238
Austen, Jane, 96

B

Baby
arrival of, 171–75
being cool with,
221–28
breastfeeding, 70–71,
181–82, 194–95,
205–9
caring for, 49, 177–85
daycare for, 131–37
excuses and, 213–16
feeding, 70–71, 181–
82, 194–95, 205–9
healthy baby, 25–31
illness of, 215–16
myths about, 237–40
nurturing, 49
preparing for, 65–73,
163–69
reflections on,
243–47
supplies for, 68,
71–72
Baby shower, 71
Bad habits, 25–31,
69–70, 76, 98
Barry, Dave, 15
Bialik, Mayim, 246

Birthing class, 153–59
Birthing room, 156–57
Birth of baby, 171–75
Birth plan, 155–56
Blaine, David, 157, 204
Bloomingdale, Theresa,
179
Body, changes in, 81–87,
163–69, 187–91
Brault, Robert, 113
Breastfeeding, 70–71,
181–82, 194–95, 205–9

C

Caffeine, 30, 180, 224
Career
child care and,
131–37
discrimination and,
128
maternity leave and,
37, 68–69, 127–30
tips for, 119–25
Carrey, Jim, 230
Chalmers, Irena, 206
Changes, in body, 81–
87, 163–69, 187–91
Changes, rolling with,
39–40
Child care options,
131–37
Cigarettes, 25–30,
69–70, 98
Clothing, maternity,
89–93

Clothing, postpartum,
199–204
Cody, Diablo, 156
Cold feet, 44–45
Cole, Jim, 155
Co-parenting, 114
Cravings, 78, 80. *See also*
Foods
Cruise, Tom, 237

D

Darrow, Clarence, 44
Daycare options, 131–37
Depp, Johnny, 56, 202
Diapers, changing,
180–81
Diapers, cost of, 70
Didion, Joan, 225
Diet, 75–80, 95–99. *See
also* Foods
Dining out, 69–70
Doctor, consulting,
26–29, 72, 76–77, 90
Doctorow, E. L., 14
Drinking, 25–30, 69–70,
76
Drugs, 25–30, 49

E

Emotions
coping with, 35–36,
101–7
crying, 103–4
jealousy, 43
repressed feelings,
101–2, 106

support group for, 105

walking and, 106–7, 190

Ephron, Nora, 158

Excuses, 36, 122, 213–16

Exercise, 98, 106–7, 190

F

Family, growing, 67, 147–51

Family, help from, 59–63, 189–90, 195

Family Medical Leave Act (FMLA), 127

Farrow, Mia, 238

Finances, 38–39, 67–72. *See also* Money

Fisher, Carrie, 106

Flash-forwards, 183–84

Focus, achieving, 40

Foods
to avoid, 75–80

healthy foods, 35, 96–98, 105

nutrition, 75–80, 95–99

raw foods, 77–79

spicy foods, 78

weight gain and, 82–83, 95–97, 105, 188–89

Free time, loss of, 139–46

Friends, 59–63, 189–90, 229–35

Frost, David, 149

G

Gaskin, Ina May, 188

Gestational diabetes, 79, 97

Gilbert, Christine, 27

Gilden, Julia, 158

Grooming, 81–87, 166

Guidance from others, 229–35

H

Health insurance, 72

Healthy baby, 25–31

Healthy foods, 35, 96–98, 105

Home
cleaning, 38, 68

relocating, 68

size of, 68

Hospital bills, 68, 72

Hudson, Kate, 190

Humor, sense of, 62, 106, 190, 224, 227

Hygiene, 81–87, 166

I

Ibuprofen, 30, 180, 224

Insurance, 72, 128–29

Ivins, Molly, 12

J

Job
child care and, 131–37

discrimination and, 128

maternity leave and, 37, 68–69, 127–30

tips for, 119–25

Jones, Catherine, 244

K

Kassis, Sandra Chami, 60

L

Labor, 154, 171–75

Life, as mother, 177–85, 187–91

Life, simplifying, 36–37

M

Maternity clothes, 89–93

Maternity leave, 37, 68–69, 127–30

Mayer, Marissa, 119

McClintock, Jessica, 199

Medical insurance, 72

Money
accumulating, 38–39, 67–70

for hospital bills, 68, 72

for living expenses, 68

for newborn care supplies, 68

saving, 38–39, 69–71

spending, 68–72

Moss, Kate, 56

Mother
caring for, 187–91

clothing for, 89–93, 199–204

excuses and, 213–16

to multiple children, 67, 147–51

new life as, 23, 177–85, 187–91, 225–27, 243–47

types of, 229–35
Motherhood, 23, 181, 225–27, 243–47
Multiple children, 67, 147–51
Myths, 237–40

N

Nursing baby, 70–71, 181–82, 194–95, 205–9
Nurturing baby, 49
Nutrition, 75–80, 95–99. *See also* Foods

O

Obstetrician, 26–27
Olinghouse, Lane, 143

P

Paltrow, Gwyneth, 45, 190
Panic, 65–66
Paranoia, 183–84
Parenthood, 23, 181, 225–27, 243–47
Parenting methods, 229–35
Picoult, Jodi, 223
Pitt, Brad, 19
Postpartum clothes, 199–204
Postpartum side effects, 174–75, 184, 189, 220
Preparing for baby, 65–73

R

Reflections, 243–47
Relationship
assessing, 39, 111–12
communication in, 111–18
counseling for, 113–15
date nights, 117
helpful tips for, 111–18
Resources, 249–51
Rickman, Alan, 183
Rockwell, Norman, 57
Rogen, Seth, 114
Rudeness, 54–56

S

Sandburg, Carl, 9
Sedaris, David, 225
Sex
post-birth sex, 217–20
during pregnancy, 86–87, 111–12
safeness of, 30
Sexton, Anne, 225
Shock, 19–23
Simpson, Jessica, 83
Sleep, lack of, 177–78, 182–83
Smith, Patti, 225
Smoking, 25–30, 69–70, 98
Social activities, 41–46
Support group, 105

T

Tucci, Stanley, 28

U

Unplanned pregnancies
advantages to, 35–40
disadvantages to, 33
explaining, 56–58
handling, 11–15
statistics on, 19–20

V

Visitors, 193–97

W

Walking, 106–7, 190
Weight gain, 82–83, 95–97, 105, 188–89
Weight loss, 173, 202–4
Weiner, Jennifer, 20
White, Jack, 224
Williams, Robin, 230
Wine, 30, 76, 99, 233–34

ABOUT THE AUTHOR

Tracy Moore is a writer in Los Angeles who loves Brussels sprouts, defending the lowbrow, and writing rabidly commented-on columns about parenting, sex, relationships, culture, and gender for the Gawker-owned ladyblog *Jezebel*. She and her husband spend all the rest of their extremely limited free time party-hopping local parks, wrangling a three-year-old who does not ever allow them to watch regular, non-cartoon TV.